AIDS &
POLITICS

All About **AIDS**

Books in This Series

AIDS & Politics
AIDS & Poverty
AIDS & Science
AIDS & Society
AIDS & You

AIDS & POLITICS

Jacquelyn Simone

AlphaHouse Publishing
New York

All About **AIDS**
AIDS & Politics

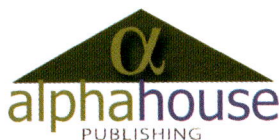

AlphaHouse Publishing
A Division of PEMG Publishing Group, Inc.
201 Harding Avenue
Vestal, New York 13850
www.alphahousepublishing.com

First Printing
9 8 7 6 5 4 3 2 1
ISBN: 978-1-934970-23-2
ISBN (set): 978-1-934970-22-5
    Library of Congress Control Number: 2008930650

Author: Simone, Jacquelyn

Cover design by Wendy Arakawa.
Interior design by MK Bassett-Harvey.

Printed in India by International Print-O-Pac Limited

An ISO 9001 Company

Contents

Introduction

What do you know about HIV/AIDS? Where do you get your information? From your friends? From your parents? At school? From television?

You hear a lot about AIDS and HIV these days. But lots of kids—and adults, too—don't really understand HIV/AIDS. They need clearly presented, straightforward facts to replace false information from family and friends and keep themselves safe.

HIV/AIDS is a global epidemic. The facts, from the World Health Organization (WHO) and UNICEF, *can be* scary:

- 33.2 million people were living with HIV/AIDS at the end of 2007.
- 290,000 children under the age of 15 died from HIV/AIDS in 2007.
- More than 2/3 of the population of sub-Saharan Africa is infected with HIV/AIDS.
- Over 15 million children under the age of 18 have lost one or both parents to AIDS, and millions more have been made vulnerable.

No matter how scary the facts seem, they should not overpower us. The world is fighting HIV/AIDS every day at the global and the individual level. There is no cure for

HIV, but there are treatments. However, many people in the world continue to go without the treatments they need. In fact, the Joint United Nations Programme on HIV/AIDS (UNAIDS) reports that, globally, less than one person in five at risk of HIV has access to basic HIV prevention services and only 31% of people who needed HIV treatment had access to it by the end of 2007. This series talks about why, and what organizations such as the WHO and UNAIDS are doing about the problem.

These books discuss the effects of different aspects of society on the HIV/AIDS pandemic. For example, gender, age, poverty, political struggles, and geography all affect peoples' overall health and access to treatment. In addition, many people, afraid of the social stigma and perceived death sentence of an HIV diagnosis, avoid seeking help when it is needed.

The truth is vital to preventing further spread of the disease. People need to get tested, learn their status, and begin antiretroviral therapy treatment in order to help prevent spreading the disease to others. Education is key to this process of prevention. This series promotes prevention and action through education. The books are intended for distribution to families, libraries, and schools around the world to help reduce fear, increase knowledge, and promote prevention.

The series also touches on what the world is doing to end the HIV/AIDS epidemic and offers suggestions for how readers can get involved at the individual, community, or global level.

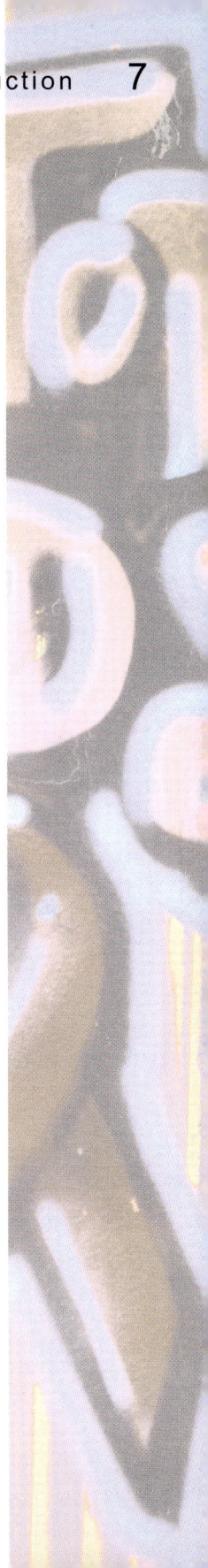

Here's what you need to know

- HIV stands for Human Immune Deficiency Virus. It's the virus that causes AIDS.
- AIDS stands for Acquired Immunodeficiency Syndrome.
- HIV/AIDS hurts your body's ability to fight off other diseases and infections.
- You CAN'T catch HIV/AIDS from touching an infected person or being around an infected person.
- The only way to catch HIV/AIDS is from an infected person's body fluids.
- You can be infected:
  - during sex.
  - by sharing dirty drug, tattoo, or piercing needles.
  - via mother-to-infant transmission.
- In the 1970s and 1980s, people caught HIV/AIDS from blood transfusions, but now blood donors are screened before they can give blood.
- Although scientists have not found a cure for HIV/AIDS, they have found better medicines that help a person with the virus live longer, with fewer symptoms.
- Scientists are still looking for either a cure or a vaccine that would keep people from getting the disease.
- HIV medicines are very expensive and not everyone can afford them.
- Poverty and HIV/AIDS are two of the biggest problems facing the world today—and they are connected to each other.

1
What Is HIV/AIDS?

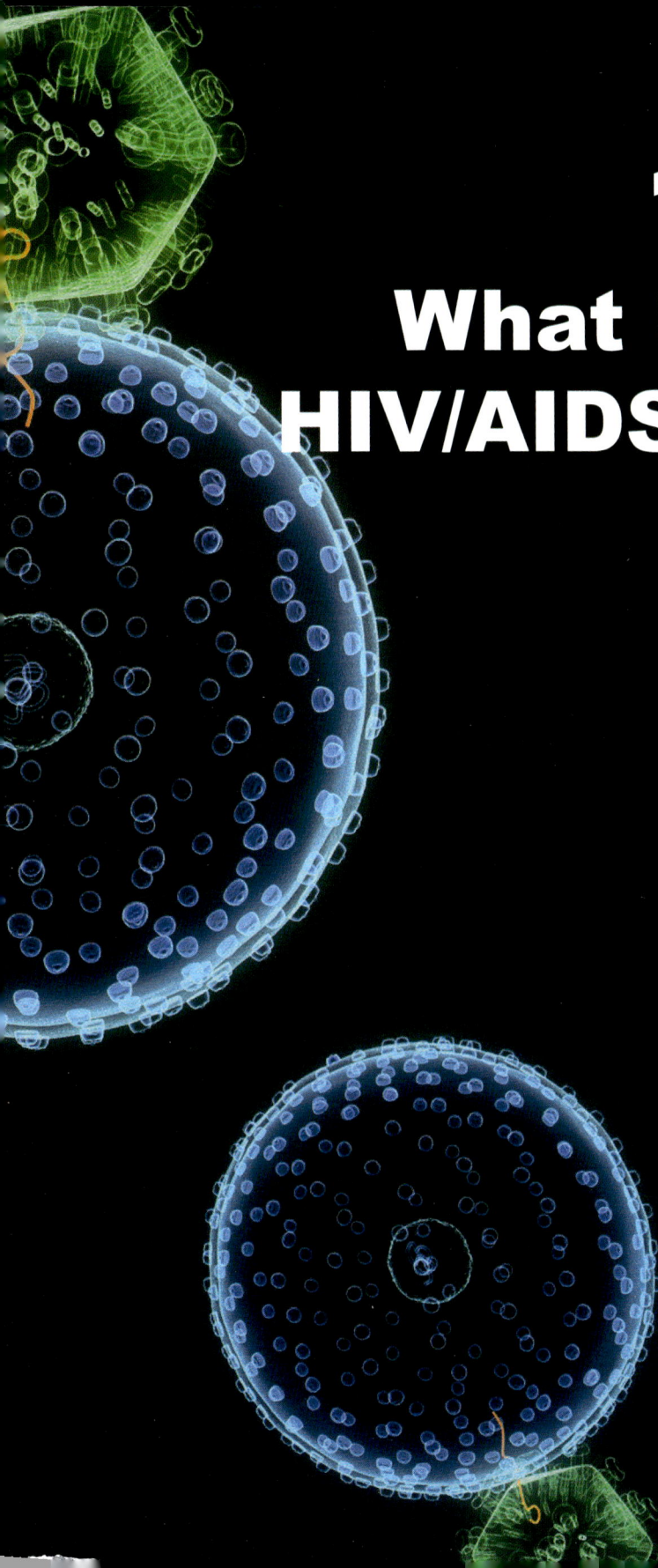

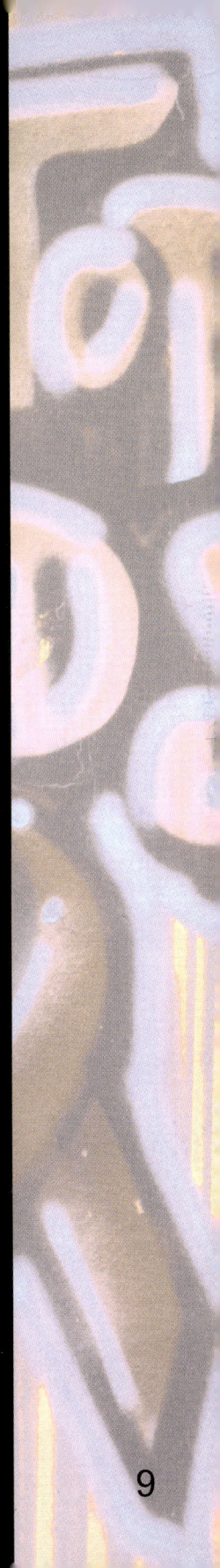

Words to Understand

If something is *acquired*, you get it through something you do (rather than it coming to you through your genes or some other part of your make-up over which you have no control).

Your *immune system* fights off germs and keeps you from getting sick.

A *deficiency* is when you don't have enough of something.

A *syndrome* is a collection of disease symptoms doctors don't completely understand.

Antibodies are special proteins in your blood that fight germs.

If something is *infectious* it can pass from one person to another.

Transfusions are injections of blood or blood components into the bloodstream.

Developed nations are countries where the majority of the population have higher incomes with all the services they need. There are many industries in these countries. Most of Japan, the United States, Canada, Israel, and many of the countries in Europe are all developed countries.

Developing nations are countries where most of the people live in poverty and have few educational, professional, and medical opportunities. Much of the population usually depends on farming for their livelihoods, and there are few industries. Most of the countries of Africa and South America are considered to be developing nations.

Crises are turning points in life. Often the outcomes of these moments are terrible—but the potential for new growth and a better world is also present in every crisis as well.

You hear a lot about AIDS and HIV these days. You've probably seen television shows and movies where characters had this disease. You hear about it at school. You may even know someone who has it. You may think it's connected somehow to homosexuals. But lots of kids—and adults too—don't really understand what HIV/AIDS is. They don't know how you catch it, who gets it, or what causes it. Lots of people don't even know what these letters stand for.

HIV stands for human immunodeficiency virus. It's the virus that causes AIDS—acquired immunodeficiency syndrome. People may have the HIV virus in their bodies and still have no symptoms that they're sick. As the disease becomes worse, though, and people develop symptoms, it often is referred to as AIDS.

Acquired immunodeficiency syndrome—AIDS—got its name because:

• It is *acquired*; in other words, it is a condition that has to be passed to you from another person. It cannot be inherited from your parents or passed along to you by your genes. This means if your boyfriend has HIV/AIDS you could catch it from him—but if your grandmother who lives in another country has HIV/AIDS, you're not going to discover that she passed it on to you.

- It affects the body's *immune* system, the part of the body that fights off diseases.
- It is considered a *deficiency* because it makes the immune system stop working the way it should.
- At first doctors thought it was a *syndrome* because people with AIDS experience a number of different symptoms and diseases. A syndrome is a word doctors use for a collection of symptoms they don't completely understand, and when the term AIDS was first used, doctors only knew about the disease's late stages. They didn't understand exactly what was making people sick. Today, doctors think that "HIV disease" is a better name, but AIDS is still the name that most people use.

Your Immune System

The worst thing about AIDS is that it hurts your immune system—the special cells in your blood that fight off germs

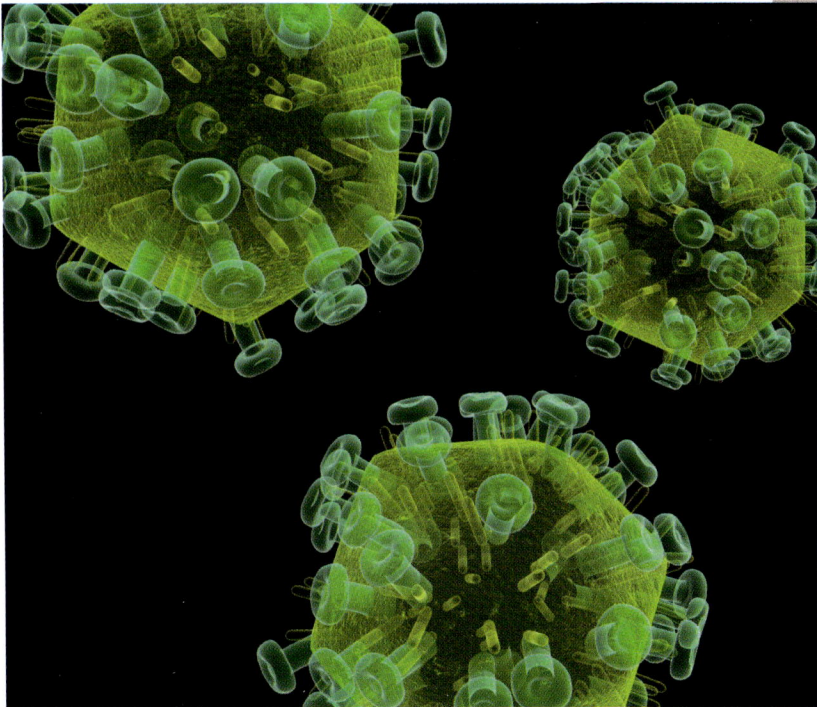

The HIV virus is a tiny organism that needs a host cell in order to act like a living thing. Unlike most living things, viruses have no cells. Instead, they are made mostly of genetic material that changes the cells they infect.

If you think you may have been exposed to the HIV virus, go to your doctor or clinic and get your blood tested. It may be scary to find out the truth—but it's better to know. Even if the news isn't good, new treatments mean that a person with HIV may often live a healthy life for a long time.

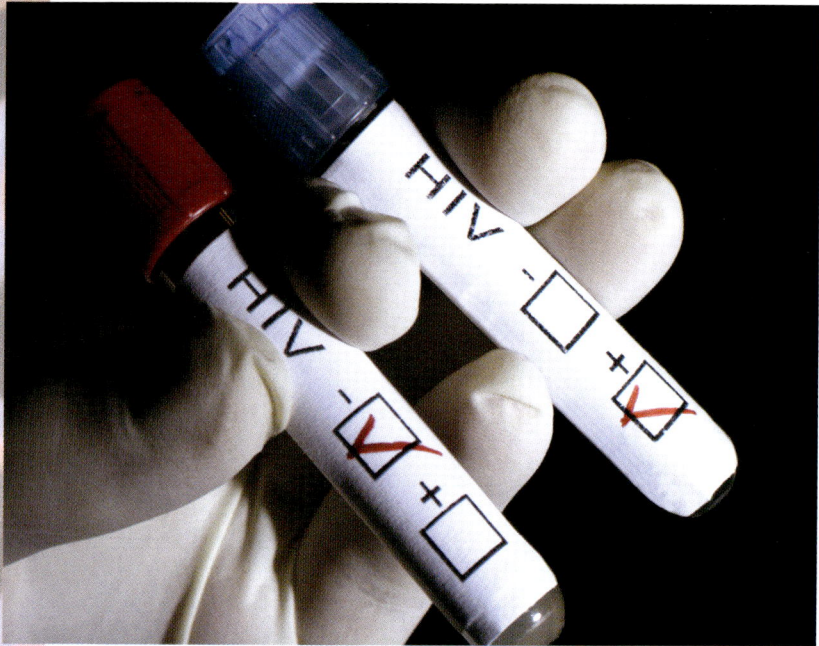

and keep you from getting sick. When this happens, you can get sick with other infections, and your body won't be able to fight off the illness. People with AIDS often actually die from another disease (such as an infection caused by a fungus, pneumonia, brain infections, or cancer).

When a virus or bacteria (what we often call germs) get into your body through a cut, through the air you breathe, or through something you've eaten, special cells in your blood, white blood cells called helper T cells, also called CD4 lymphocytes, get busy. They pass along the message to another group of white blood cells—B cells—telling them to make the weapons (called *antibodies*) they need to kill the germs. If a virus or bacteria makes its way past the antibodies, it can cause an infection. When that happens, a different type of T cell recognizes the change in the infected cell and kills it. This prevents the infection from spreading. At least this is what is *supposed* to happen.

When someone has HIV, eventually she will no longer be able to fight off infections that other people have no problem resisting. As HIV grows within her body, her immune system gets weaker and weaker. She will become more ill more often, especially with certain kinds of cancer and pneumonia.

Doctors say that a person has AIDS when:

- he has tested positive for HIV in his blood.
- he has had one or more AIDS-related infections or illnesses.
- the number of CD4 lymphocytes has reached or fallen below 200 per cubic millimeter of blood (a healthy person's T-cell count ranges between 450 and 1,200).

A few people will have AIDS within a few months from the time they are first exposed to HIV, but that's not usual. In most people, symptoms do not show up for ten to twelve years. It's very important to find out if a person has HIV as soon as possible, because doctors now have medicines that can make most people go even longer before developing AIDS.

The Spread of HIV/AIDS

This table shows how many people were living with AIDS in different parts of the world in 2004, compared to 3 years earlier.

Region	2001	2004
Sub-Sahara Africa	23.8 million	25.4 million
South & Southeast Asia	5.9 million	6.4 million
Latin American	1.4 million	1.7 million
Eastern & Central Europe	890,000	1.4 million
East Asia & Pacific	680,000	1.1 million
North America	950,000	1 million
Western Europe	540,000	610,000
North Africa & Middle East	340,000	540,000
Caribbean	400,000	440,000
Oceania	24,000	35,000

In the years since 2004, the numbers have continued to climb.

Did You Know?

Scientists and doctors gave HIV/AIDS its name in the 1980s when the first people started getting sick with it. At the beginning, many patients were homo- sexual men— which made some people think this was a "homosexual problem"—but before long, doctors realized other people were getting sick with HIV and AIDS too. AIDS is an "everybody" problem.

The one to three months after a person is first infected with the HIV virus is when that person is most *infec- tious*. The amount of virus in her system is at its highest and T-cell counts are at their lowest, which means she is most likely to pass along the disease to others. During this time, her body has not had time to react to the virus and produce the cells that will fight the virus. Meanwhile, the virus is reproducing itself within the body.

You can't tell that all this is happening. On the out- side, there are no symptoms, and a person who is infected can look and feel perfectly well for many years; he may not even know he is infected. As the immune system gets weaker, however, the person becomes more likely to catch the illnesses that the immune system would normally have been able to fight. As time goes by, he is more likely to become ill more often and develop AIDS.

How Does HIV Spread?

First, how does it *not* spread? HIV CANNOT be spread by:

- shaking hands with someone who has HIV/AIDS
- hugging someone who has HIV/AIDS
- sharing eating utensils with someone who has HIV/AIDS

Scientists have found that the HIV virus can survive in needles for more than a month. This means that if you inject drugs with a used needle, you may be shooting HIV into your bloodstream!

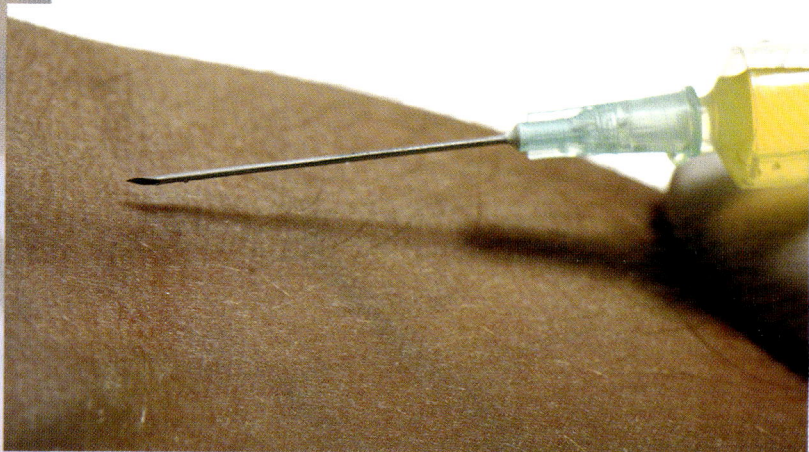

Real People

Ryan White began 1984 as a typical thirteen-year-old. He had hemophilia, but it was being treated. He went to school and had friends, just like most kids his age. Then Ryan and his family found out he had caught HIV through the blood products he had received to treat his hemophilia. The HIV had already advanced to AIDS. Doctors told Ryan and his family that he only had six months to live.

Ryan wanted to spend the last months of his life doing what he had been doing, going to school and being with friends. But the school didn't want him there. People were afraid Ryan's illness might "rub off" on the other students. Ryan's battle to be allowed to attend school made news first in the United States and then all over the world. Because of Ryan, people all over the world started thinking about AIDS.

On April 8, 1990, Ryan White lost his battle with AIDS. He was only nineteen when he died, but he had done a lot with his life. Because he fought hard to make people realize that AIDS is a problem we must all face, laws were passed to help people with HIV/AIDS, television shows were made, magazine articles were written, and education programs were started in schools. The world began to work together to fight this terrible disease—all because one young boy was brave enough to take a stand.

• being in the same room with someone who has HIV/AIDS
• touching something that someone with HIV/AIDS has touched
• breathing the same air as someone with HIV/AIDS

Doctors have never found any cases where someone caught HIV by doing any of these things with a family member, friend, or coworker.

The ONLY way to become infected with HIV is through certain body fluids. The person infected with the virus carries it in blood, semen, vaginal secretions, and breast milk. In order for you to catch HIV, one of these fluids from a person with HIV would have to enter your bloodstream. Here are the most common ways that HIV could get into your blood:

• during unprotected sex (sex where no condom is used)
• during the kind of drug use where the user "shoots up" with a needle (if the needle is dirty and was used by someone who has HIV)
• through a cut or sore on the skin.

The most common way to catch HIV is through unprotected sexual intercourse. This means any kind of sex—oral, anal, or vaginal. Women are more at risk for catching HIV

Global Statistics on HIV/AIDS

Number of people living with HIV

Adults	38.0 million
Women	17.5 million
Children under age 15	2.3 million
Total	40.3 million

People Newly Infected with HIV
(according to UN and WHO research)

Adults	4.2 million
Children under age 15	700,000
Total	4.9 million

AIDS Deaths

Adults	2.6 million
Children under age 15	570,000
Total	3.1 million

this way than are their male partners, but women can also pass along HIV to men through sexual intercourse.

Some drug users share needles and other equipment. This makes intravenous drug users another group of people who often get HIV. Needles used for body piercing and tattooing can also carry HIV and should not be reused. If you decide to get a piercing or a tattoo, be sure to only have it done by someone who uses only clean equipment.

The youngest people with AIDS—the babies—generally get the disease from their mothers. In most of these cases, the mother does not know she is infected, especially since there can be many years between when she was exposed to the virus and when she first gets symptoms. If there is any chance a woman has been exposed to HIV, she should be tested for the virus before becoming pregnant. Medicine can be given to pregnant women with HIV to protect to their babies during pregnancy. After the baby is

Researchers are developing new medicines that are more effective at fighting the HIV virus. Unfortunately, some of the areas of the world that need this medication most are too poor to afford it.

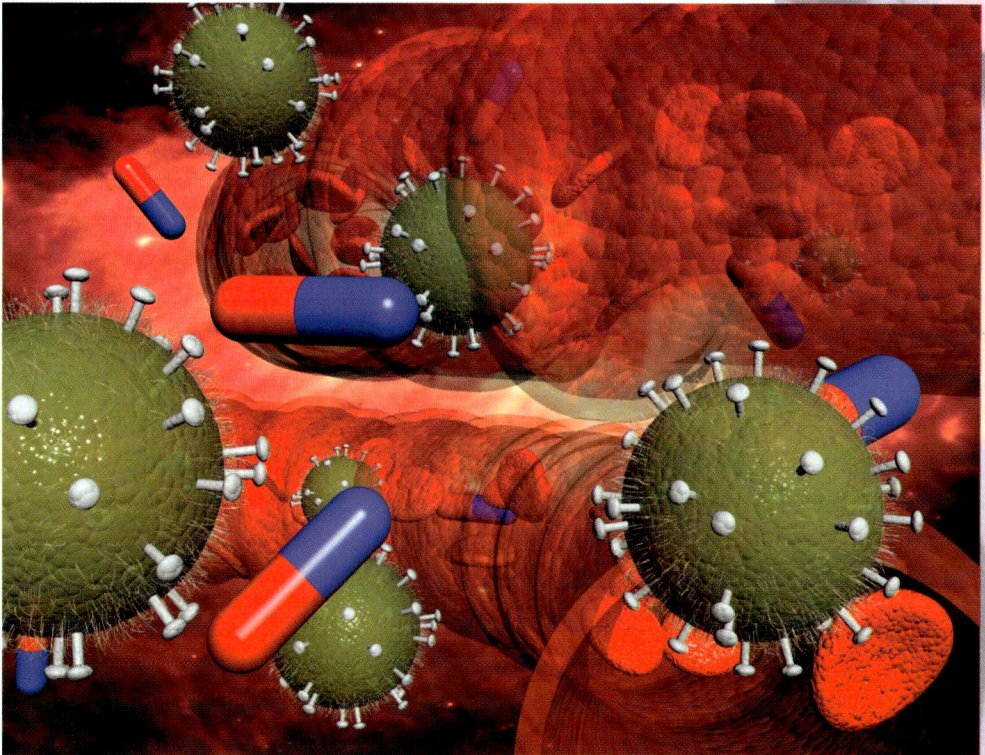

born, women with HIV should not breastfeed, so that the virus isn't passed to their babies through breast milk.

HIV/AIDS and Blood Transfusions

In the 1970s and early 1980s, before anyone knew very much about HIV/AIDS, blood donors who didn't know they had the disease gave their blood to hospitals and at Red Cross blood drives—and the virus got into the blood supply that was given out to sick or injured people who needed blood *transfusions*. Eventually, doctors realized that some people were catching HIV/AIDS from blood transfusions. Beginning in 1985, the blood supply has been tested for HIV, and there is no longer much risk that someone will get HIV/AIDS from a blood transfusion. However, people who received transfusions between 1975 and 1985 had a high risk of receiving infected blood. Among those most at risk were people with hemophilia.

Hemophilia

Hemophilia is an illness in which blood clots much more slowly than normal. As a result, small cuts and other injuries can cause heavy bleeding. Boys are more apt to have this disease than girls.

Using a condom is one of the best ways to protect yourself against the HIV virus.

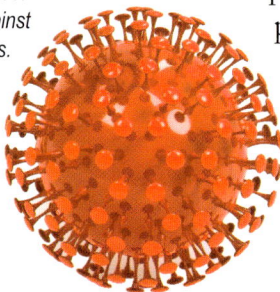

People with hemophilia must use blood and blood products to control bleeding episodes. This made them vulnerable to the contaminated blood supply between 1975 and 1985. Some reports indicate that during this time, as many as half of the individuals with hemophilia were infected with HIV through blood and blood products. According to the Web site www.hivpositive.com, an estimated 10,000 people with hemophilia have HIV today.

You cannot get HIV by donating blood. And today, the risk of becoming infected with HIV through the use of blood and blood

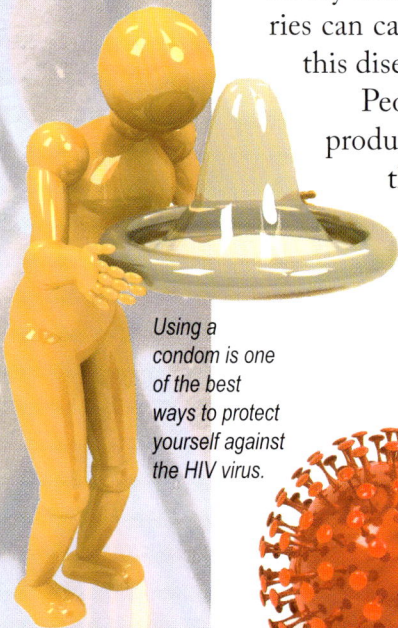

products is greatly reduced for individuals with hemophilia. More careful screening of blood donors has been one reason for this; blood from every donor is checked for HIV before it is used. New methods of treating the blood and blood products, including the use of heat, have also reduced the risk.

Treatment for HIV/AIDS

Up until recently, if you found out you had HIV, you thought you would die soon. Today, however, some people who have the virus have still not developed AIDS even after many years. AIDS has no cure yet, but many people with HIV are living longer and staying healthier. New medicines have made this possible.

For many people living with HIV/AIDS, a single medicine does not work. Most take a combination of many drugs,

HIV does not respond well to just one single medicine. Instead, doctors have found that the disease responds best to a combination of various medicines. Taking so many pills can be hard to remember —and it's expensive.

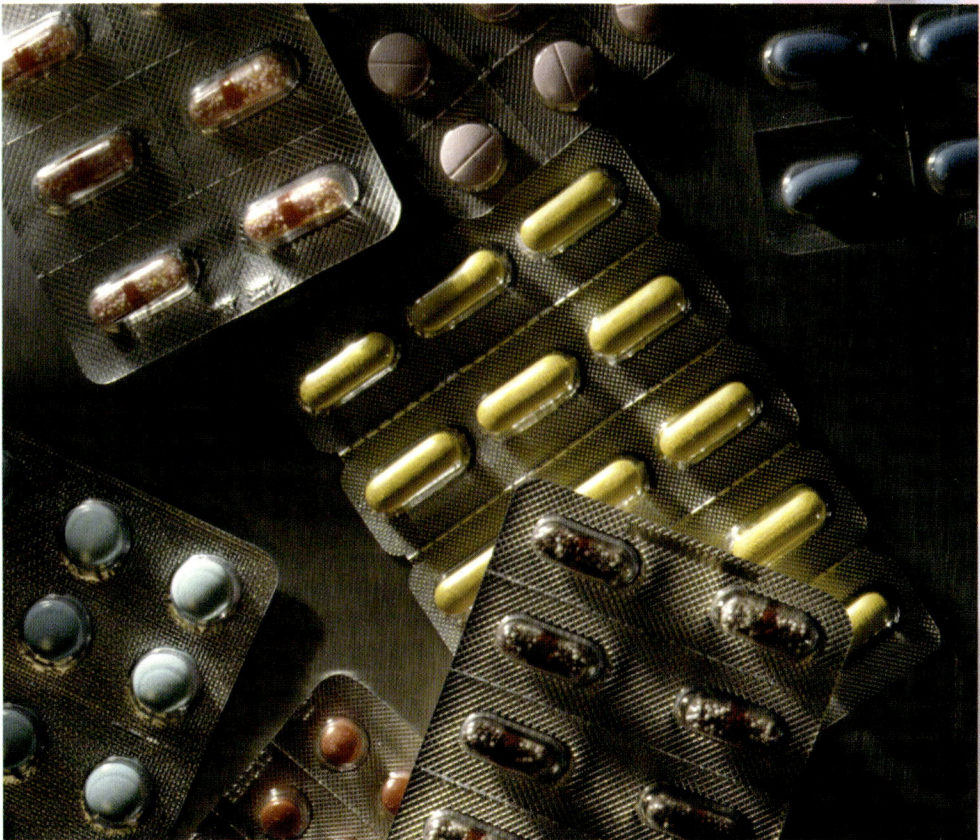

A global view of HIV infection
39.5 million people [34.1-47.1] living with HIV in 2006

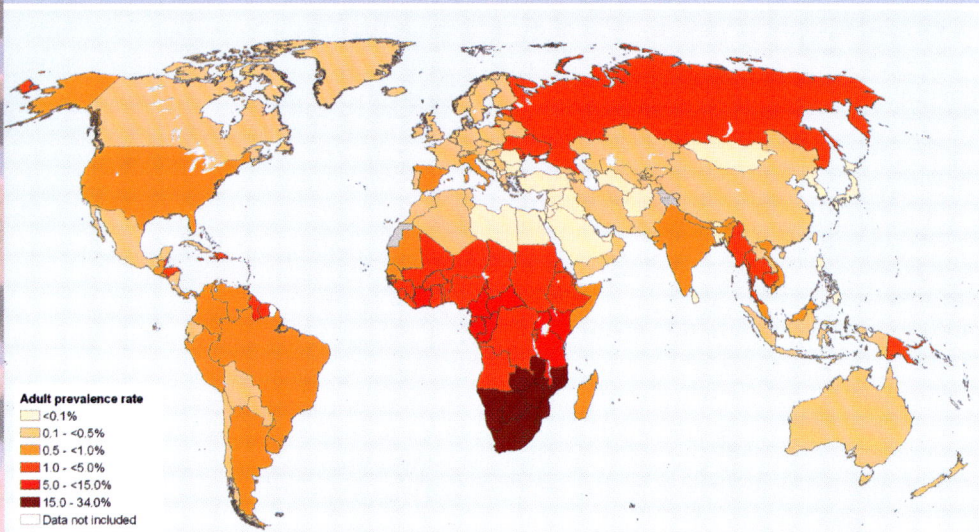

Adult prevalence rate
- <0.1%
- 0.1 - <0.5%
- 0.5 - <1.0%
- 1.0 - <5.0%
- 5.0 - <15.0%
- 15.0 - 34.0%
- Data not included

The boundaries and names shown and the designations used on this map do not imply the expression of any opinion whatsoever on the part of the World Health Organization concerning the legal status of any country, territory, city or area or of its authorities, or concerning the delimitation of its frontiers or boundaries. Dotted lines on maps represent approximate border lines for which there may not yet be full agreement.

Data Source: WHO / UNAIDS
Map Production: Public Health Mapping and GIS
Communicable Diseases (CDS)
World Health Organization

World Health Organization

sometimes called a "cocktail." The medicines have to be taken a certain way at certain times in order for them to work. They work together to reduce the level of HIV in the body, allowing the body's own CD4 lymphocytes to return to healthier levels. This is good news. But it doesn't mean that HIV/AIDS is no longer a huge problem in our world today.

For one thing, some people have a hard time remembering when and how to take so many different kinds of medicines. Imagine if you had to take four or more different pills every day at different times throughout the day. You'd probably forget sometimes. So do lots of people who are taking these medicines. But when they do, the medicines don't work as well for them, and new forms of the virus can develop.

The medicines also have some bad side effects. They can damage a person's kidneys, heart, and bones. If this happens, the person cannot keep taking the medicines.

But the worst problem with these medicines is that they are very expensive. Around the world, many of the people living with HIV/AIDS are also living in poverty. They may have no money to buy the medicines or even go to the doctor. They may live in a region so poor that they don't even have a doctor or clinic nearby where they could go if they did have money.

People living with HIV/AIDS in North America, Europe, and other *developed nations* have a better chance of living longer, even when they are poor. Many of these countries have special programs to help bring AIDS medicines to people living in poverty. These programs are not perfect; many times people may make just enough money that they don't qualify, but not enough money that they can afford to buy the medicines on their own. But as researchers find new ways to treat HIV/AIDS, these people may one day have access to better medicine and even a vaccine.

Some of the world's *developing nations* don't have even the most basic medicines to treat their people, let

These hands belong to poor children in Ethiopia. Their risk of contracting HIV is high, and poverty makes their situation worse.

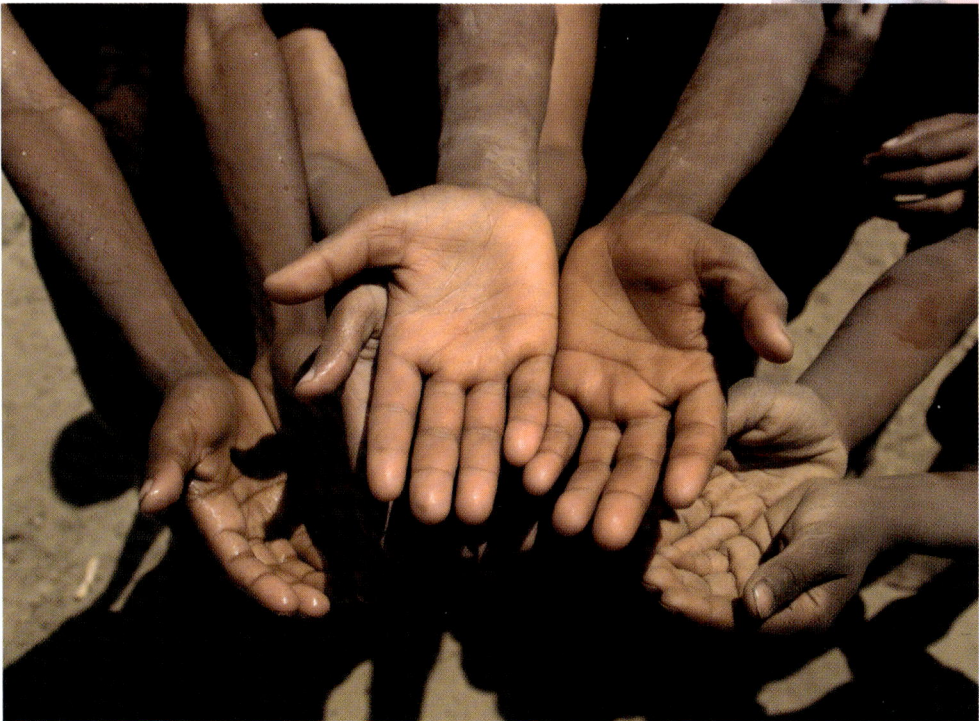

How Can You Keep Yourself Safe?

The only way to be sure you won't catch HIV/AIDS is to protect yourself from other people's body fluids. Sex is the way most people come into contact with body fluids. So if you don't want to catch HIV/AIDS, you need to protect yourself by not having sex until you are sure it is safe. Women and men don't need to worry about getting HIV/AIDS from each other:

- if neither partner ever had sex with anyone else.

- if neither partner ever shared needles.

- if neither partner currently has or ever had HIV/AIDS.

What Is Safer Sex?

The only way to be absolutely certain you don't catch something from a sexual partner is to not have sex until you know you're in safe relationship where both of you will keep your promises to be faithful to each other. However, "safer sex" is anything you can do to lower your risk of getting HIV/AIDS (or another disease) if you do choose to have sex outside a safe relationship. The most important ways to reduce your risk are:

- Keep your partner's body fluids out of your body, including your vagina, anus, or mouth. The body fluids to be most careful about are blood, semen, vaginal fluids, and the runny discharge from sores.

Safer sex also means protecting your partner:

- Don't allow your body fluids to get into your partner's body.

- Don't have sex if you have sores or other symptoms of infection.

- Have routine checkups for sexually transmitted infections.

- Get the correct treatment if you become infected.

When you are a child, it's the job of the adults in your life to protect you and keep you safe. As you get older, though, it will be up to you to protect yourself from danger. Take care of yourself! Make sure you're not one of the millions of people around the world who are living with HIV/AIDS.

along the medications that treat HIV/AIDS. Sometimes the nation's government controls the medicines, and the government decides who gets the medicine, often based on how much money the person has. The big companies that make the medicines are also part of the problem. Sometimes these companies have refused to sell drugs at lower prices to the developing world.

Poverty and AIDS are enormous *crises* in today's world, both in developed and developing countries. You can't separate them from each other—poverty makes AIDS a bigger problem, and AIDS makes poverty a bigger problem. We have to understand each side of the problem—and we have to fight them both.

Ask the Doctor

Q: My boyfriend and I are careful when we have sex. He always makes sure he pulls out before he comes. My older sister says I can't get pregnant if he does this. Does it also mean I wouldn't catch AIDS from him if he had it?

No! This is not a safe way to protect yourself against either pregnancy or a sexually transmitted disease like HIV/AIDS. During sexual intercourse, a man's penis has a little bit of semen on it even before he ejaculates (or "comes"). Although this is a very small amount, it is enough that you could possibly become pregnant—or get HIV/AIDS from him if he is infected. Latex condoms are the only birth-control method that can also help protect you from HIV/AIDS and other infections. And remember—use condoms correctly with water-based lubricants, to reduce the chance that they could break.

STRAIGHT FROM THE SOURCE

(From the 2004 World Health Organization (WHO) document Protecting Young People from HIV and AIDS.)

Measures to reduce the vulnerability of young people and to reduce risk are complementary and part of a continuum. In terms of the sexual transmission of HIV this is well expressed as:

❑ DELAY—your first sexual experience,

❑ REDUCE—the number of your sexual partners,

❑ PROTECT—yourself and your partner by using a condom.

This approach encourages those who are at no or low risk to remain safe, and encourages all others to move in the direction of greater safety. It helps to create a climate where adolescents can more easily delay the onset of sexual experience, which is the only 100% effective way of avoiding HIV. It addresses the need to reduce the number of sexual partners, since risks rise rapidly with multiple partners. It emphasizes the need for consistent and correct use of condoms. Without condoms, those young people who do not succeed in abstaining are left unprotected at very high risk, and there would be little prospect of reducing HIV levels in the community. Millions of young people would be left to their fate, including girls who are powerless to abstain because sex is forced or coerced. Promoting abstinence and promoting condoms are not alternatives—but complementary parts of an effective approach. Condom use is promoted in order to protect those who are having sex, not to undermine those who are not.

What Do You Think?

- According to this WHO document, what is the only 100 percent effective way to avoid HIV?

- Why do you think the chances of getting HIV go up the more times you have sex with a different person?

- Why do you think some people object to teaching kids about how to use condoms?

- Why do you think other people object to only teaching kids about "abstinence" (not having sex at all)?

- What approach is WHO recommending in this document regarding the condom-abstinence question?

Find Out More

To find out more about HIV/AIDS check out these Web sites:

The AIDS Handbook: Written for Middle School Kids by Middle School Kids
www.eastchester.k12.ny.us/schools/ms/AIDS/AIDS1.html

Let's Talk: Children, Families, and HIV
www.kidstalkaids.org/education/index.html

YouthAIDS (What You Can Do to Change the World)
www.youthaids.org

Here's what you need to know

- Politics deals with the distribution of resources and maintenance of order.
- Political systems include democracy, monarchy, oligarchy, and dictatorship.
- Most politicians are wealthy, and rich people hold more political power than poor people.
- Many nations have government agencies that deal with health issues.
- Universal health care, in which the government ensures that all citizens have adequate health insurance, is found in many developed nations.

Words to Understand

Governments are the forms or systems of rule from which a group of people receive direction.

Policy means a definite course of action pursued by a government.

Resources refer to the collective wealth and assets of a country.

Institutions are organizations, establishments, foundations, or societies centered around a certain cause.

Legislation refers to a law or body of laws enacted.

Elite refers to a group of people who are considered superior to others.

The *economy* has to do with the system in place for exchanging goods and services.

Capitalism is an economic system in which private individuals and corporations own the means of production and distribution and make their own economic decisions without much government involvement.

Universal health care means that everyone, without exception, receives free medical treatment within a nation.

2
What Are Politics?

You may think that politics refers to the White House or Parliament, important people wearing suits. You may have heard that it is impolite to discuss politics in certain situations, because many people have very strong and differing opinions. However, politics means much more than all of these images.

Politics refers to the process of who gets what and how. People create **governments** to make these decisions and enforce **policy** in the form of laws. Politicians determine who receives what **resources** and how those resources are used. The term is most commonly used to describe state or country governments, but politics are also observable in any human **institution**, such as a workplace or school.

When people interact, as we do constantly in everyday life, there are usually power divisions within our relationships. In most human institutions, a few people make rules and decisions for the rest of society. Their choices determine what everyone can and cannot do. Sometimes, these rules become formally enforced laws. If people do not obey the law, they are punished and might have to pay money or go to jail. In this way, laws help maintain order in society.

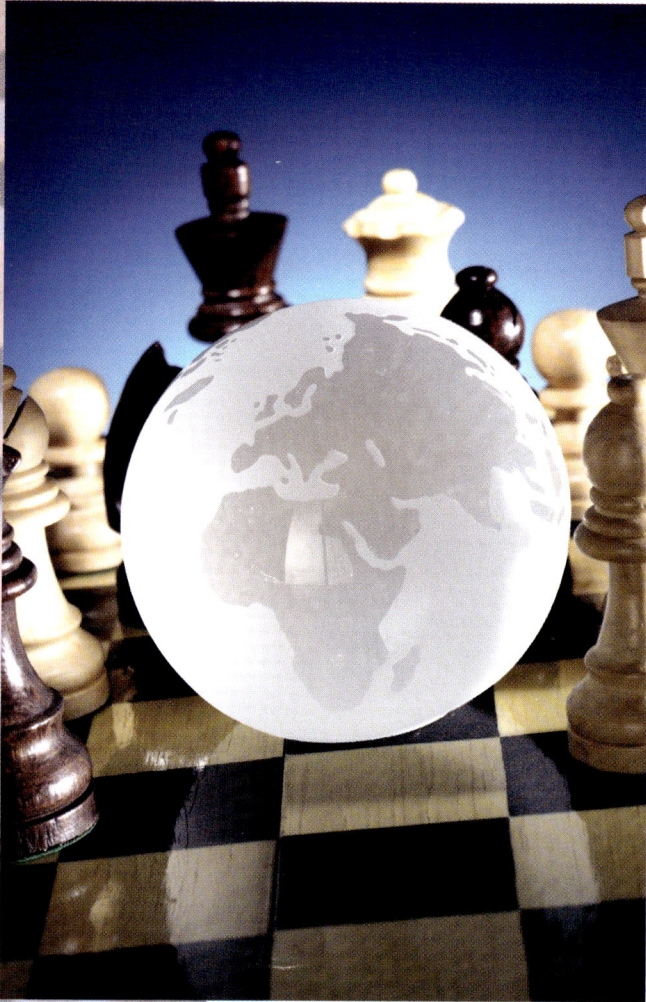

Like a game of chess, politics is made up of a set of rules that governs the world, allowing each person in a society to behave in a certain way. And like chess, the "bigger," richer players generally have more power than the smaller pawns.

The History of Politics

Politics are a part of modern society, but politics have been around for centuries. Our earliest records of human groups show that people began to organize themselves and establish governments thousands of years ago. People usually want a system of order; imagine how confusing life would be if we had no laws and people could do whatever they wanted without punishment!

Many of our modern political institutions are based on those early governments. For example, the Ancient Greeks in Athens established a system of direct democracy as early as 594 BCE. This means that all male citizens directly voted on every issue and agreed upon a set of rules. Although many countries today have a representative democracy (in

Did You Know?

According to the Institute of Medicine of the National Academy of Sciences, the U.S. is the only wealthy, developed nation that lacks universal health care.

The ancient Greeks enriched the world forever with their art, architecture, philosophy, and politics. Many people today see the Greek Acropolis as a monument to democracy.

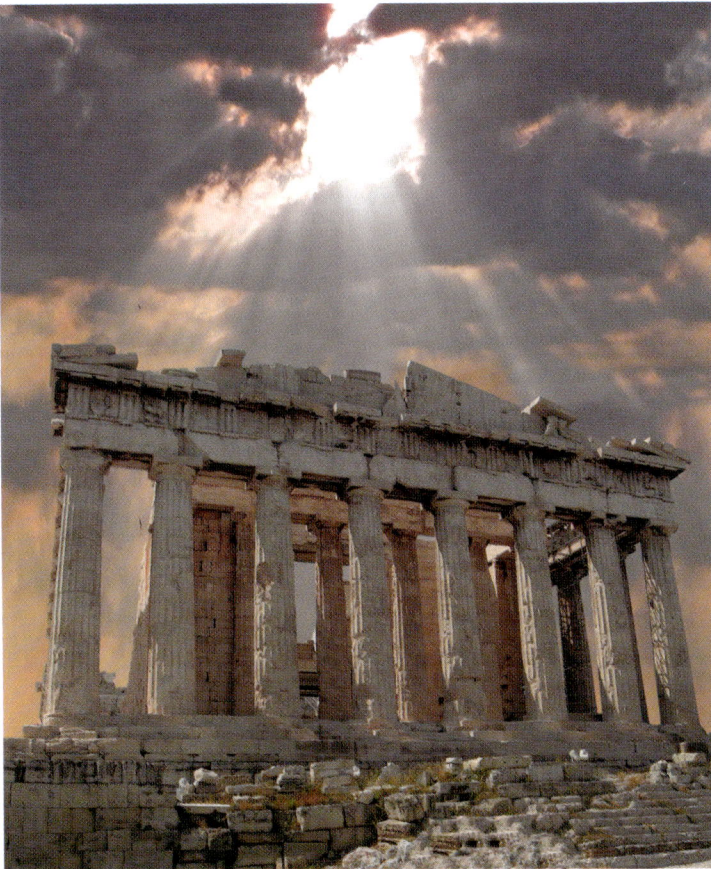

which citizens vote for people who will then vote for *legislation* in the best interests of all citizens), they borrowed the idea of democracy from the Greeks.

Not all people choose their leaders. In some countries, power is passed from generation to generation, so that only people related to the leader can ever achieve a high position. This is called a monarchy, and it was very common in Europe through the nineteenth century. Since citizens had no say in who led their country, they did not have the opportunity to select a candidate that best reflected their beliefs and opinions. When monarchs became cruel or passed a series of unpopular laws, citizens began to revolt and overthrew the monarchy, which is why there are few such government systems today.

In an oligarchy, a group of people makes all of the decisions for the rest of the country. The members of this group are usually considered socially *elite* because of their families, wealth, or military powers. An example of this system is South Africa in the twentieth century, where the people who held power were the white people, who made up only about 20 percent of the population.

Another common system is a dictatorship, in which one leader controls all power and does not usually listen to the opinions of others when making laws. Dictators can come to power through legal means, such as when Adolf Hit-

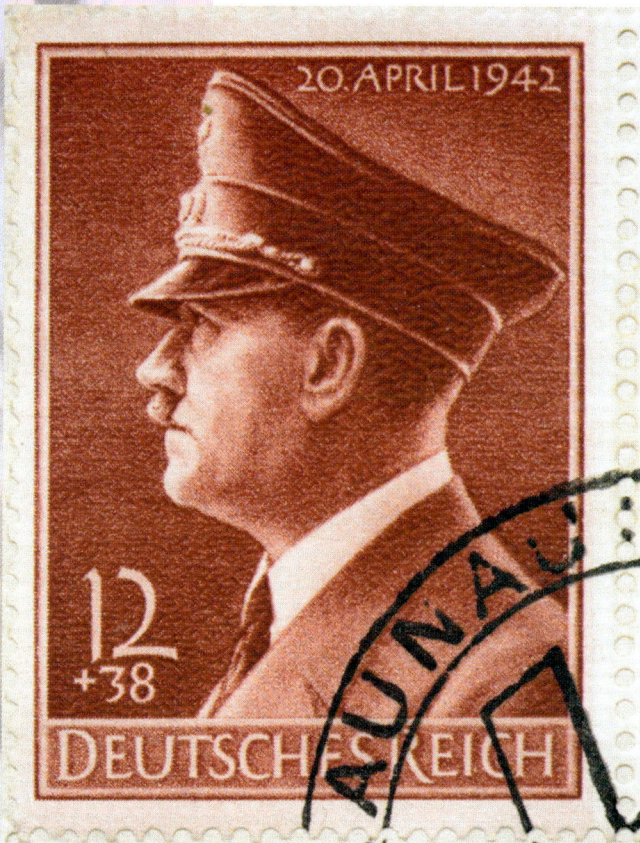

Adolf Hitler, commemorated here on this 1942 stamp, was a dictator who led his nation to commit hideous crimes against humanity—and yet he came to power legally, appointed by Germany's Chancellor. His dictatorship is an example of the great evil that politics can create.

ler was appointed Chancellor of Germany in 1933, or by seizing power illegally, as Benito Mussolini did in Italy in 1922. In monarchies, oligarchies, and dictatorships, common citizens do not have the right to elect their leaders and are therefore separated from political institutions.

Political Power

Every country has its own way of organizing the government, but almost all nations' politics have one thing in common: political power is usually determined by how much money a person has. This is especially true in countries such as the United States that encourage a type of *economy* called *capitalism*. This economic system encourages competition, so that certain people succeed and earn a lot of money while others do not. (Capitalism is the opposite of communism, in which the government controls the economy and limits economic competition.) Since it costs thousands or millions of dollars to successfully run for a political office in the United States, the people who succeed in the capitalist system are the ones who usually win in elections. The cost of advertising and travel make it nearly impossible for the average citizen to successfully compete for political office, especially on the national level.

Political Power and Health

Since politicians and people with power determine who receives benefits and resources, politics plays a large role in the area of health. Politicians decide how much assistance to give to people who cannot afford their needed medications, and they also decide how to best

Ask the Doctor

Q: I know that the United States does not have universal health care, but my grandmother tells me that the government helps her pay for her prescriptions. How is this different from universal health care?

Your grandmother is most likely covered by Medicare, the nation's largest health insurance program. Medicare, which is administered by the Centers for Medicare and Medicaid Services, covers nearly 40 million Americans. This is different from universal health care because not all citizens are covered under this program. In order to receive government assistance through Medicare, a person must be age 65 or older, disabled, or have permanent kidney failure treated with dialysis or a transplant. A related program is Medicaid, which helps certain people from low-income households pay for some of their medical bills. These programs are jointly funded by both the state and federal governments, and they are managed by the states.

create prevention programs so that other people are not infected with the disease.

The relationship between poverty and HIV/AIDS and other illnesses means that wealthy politicians might not sufficiently address such health issues. Medical bills can be very expensive, and some countries have a system of state-funded health care. This means that the government pays for hospital bills, medications, and other health-related costs. Countries such as Cuba, Canada, and the United Kingdom have such policies, which make health care affordable for all citizens. However, this system, which has often been called "socialized medicine" because of the large role of the government, might require people to pay higher taxes. Americans, for example, have often resisted paying higher taxes, and the fact that the citizens

The government of the United States is a democracy, and it intentionally patterned the architecture of its Capitol Building after the Ancient Greeks' to symbolize its ideals. Wealth and power often shape even the most idealistic of nations, however.

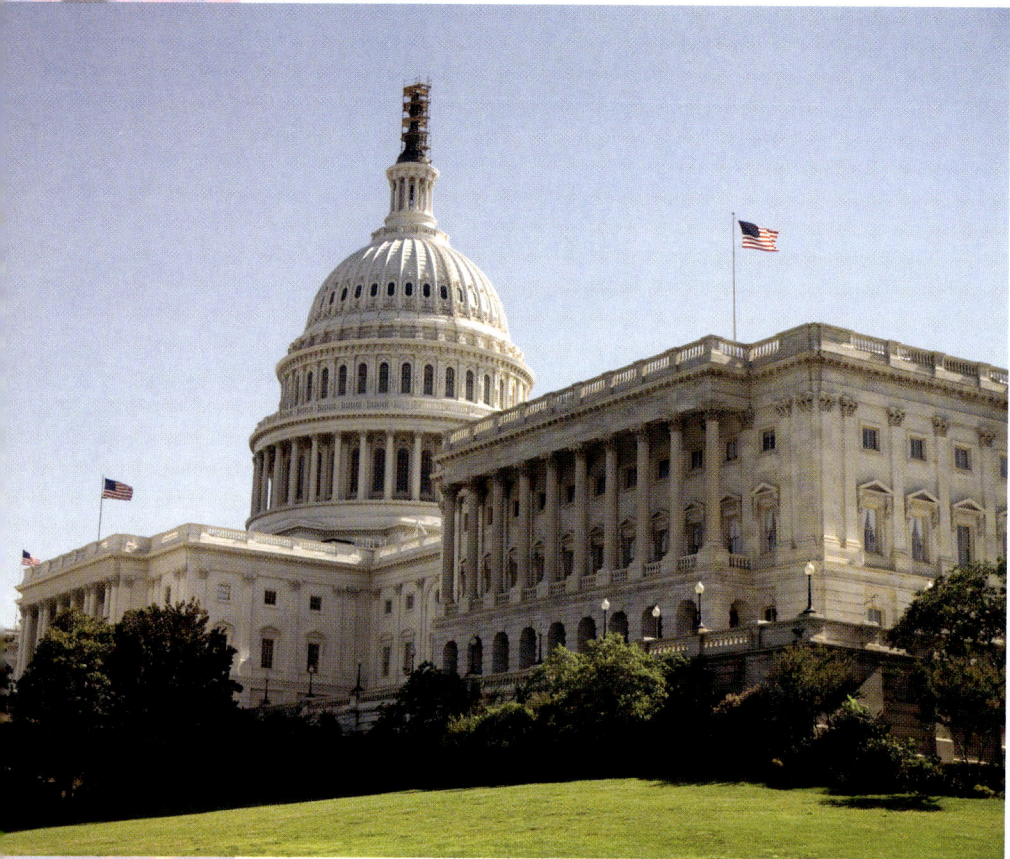

Real People

When Harvey Milk won the 1977 election to become a member of the San Francisco Board of Supervisors, he became one of the first openly gay politicians elected to office. Milk received support from the large gay population of San Francisco, but he faced frequent discrimination and death threats from more conservative citizens. While in office, he passed a law forbidding "anti-gay discrimination" in the workplace and a law requiring dog owners to clean up after their pets.

He probably would have passed more laws had his life not been cut short. On November 27, 1978, the recently resigned city supervisor Dan White shot and killed both Milk and Mayor George Moscone. White, an anti-gay conservative, received a relatively mild sentence for the murders. Milk was killed before much was known about HIV/AIDS, and there is no evidence that he had the disease. Still, the struggles he faced as a politician reveal the prejudice and homophobia in many governments. Since many politicians still see HIV/AIDS as a "gay disease," these prejudices have impacted the decisions they make about dealing with the disease.

are able to elect their representatives has prevented politicians from risking their popularity and voting in favor of *universal health care*.

When it comes to issues that involve those who live in poverty, such as AIDS, if politicians come from the wealthiest part of society, will they be able to relate to poor citizens? Does money speak louder than the voices of those who are dying from this disease?

STRAIGHT FROM THE SOURCE

(From "The Case for Universal Health Care," 2007 American Medical Student Association document.)

The Moral Case for Universal Health Care

At its root, the lack of health care for all in America is fundamentally a moral issue. The United States is the only industrialized nation that does not have some form of universal health care (defined as a basic guarantee of health care to all of its citizens). While other countries have declared health care to be a basic right, the United States treats health care as a privilege, only available to those who can afford it. In this sense, health care in America is treated as an economic good like a TV or VCR, not as a social or public good.

The Uninsured

The most visible victims of America's decision to treat health care as a privilege are the 45 million Americans who lack insurance. In contrast to prevailing stereotypes, 80% of the uninsured are hardworking Americans who are employed or come from working families. However, they are unable to obtain insurance through their work either because their employer does not offer it, their employer does offer it but the employer share of the premium is too expensive, or they are not eligible for health insurance (e.g., they are part-time or have not worked long enough at the job).

What Do You Think?

- How is universal health care defined in this document?

- Why does the author support universal health care?

- What does this document say about American priorities?

- Why do you think the United States does not guarantee health care to all citizens?

Find Out More

To find out more about poverty, check out these Web sites:

Causes of Poverty
www.globalissues.org/TradeRelated/Poverty.asp

U.S. Census Bureau, Poverty in the United States
www.census.gov/hhes/www/poverty/poverty.html

World Poverty
www.poverty.com

Here's what you need to know

- When people don't understand a disease, like the Black Death, they often panic or blame a *scapegoat*.
- Governments used to use quarantine, banishment, and killing to deal with diseases, but concerns about human rights shifted the focus to funding research.
- Today, most countries have programs to fund research and monitor national health, such as the Department of Health and Human Services and the Centers for Disease Control in the U.S. and the Canadian Institutes of Health Research.
- The United Nations was formed to promote international cooperation after World War II.
- The World Health Organization was created from the UN to provide aid for health-related issues on a global scale.
- Vaccinations have helped combat many diseases, but people in developing nations do not always have access to the vaccinations they need.

Words to Understand

A *scapegoat* is a person or group made to bear the blame for others or suffer in their place.

Epidemic diseases affect many people at the same time and are widespread in many areas.

Pandemic diseases are infectious diseases that spread across large geographic regions, such as a continent or even worldwide.

Infectious means that a disease can be spread from one person to another.

Quarantine is strict isolation that is supposed to prevent the spread of disease.

Banishment is the state of being forced to leave an area or driven away.

Globalization is an economic, political, and social trend of interconnectedness and bonds between many nations.

Mortality is the death rate.

3

Historical Perspectives on Health and Politics

Did You Know?

Most victims of the Plague died within four to seven days of infection, and four out of five people who contracted the disease died within eight days.

The Bubonic Plague—also called the Black Death—caused dark swellings on the body. In the Middle Ages, prayer and burning incense was about all that could be offered to help victims of this disease.

Throughout history, societies and governments have had to find answers for the problems faced by their citizens—and disease is an ongoing problem human beings face. Not only have political organizations been held responsible for funding treatment and research, but they also have to make sure that citizens do not panic when faced with *epidemics*. These tasks have been especially difficult when people faced or widespread diseases.

Hundreds of years ago, one of the first major diseases humanity encountered was the Bubonic Plague, or the Black Death. This disease afflicted so many people that it was a *pandemic*, meaning that it was an *infectious* disease that spread across a large region, such as a continent. Starting in the 1340s, this disease killed more than 75 million people; between 30 and 60 percent of Europe's population died.

Since people who contracted the Black Death had buboes, or black blotches caused by internal bleeding, other members of society could identify who was infected. People panicked. Often their beliefs about life and reli-

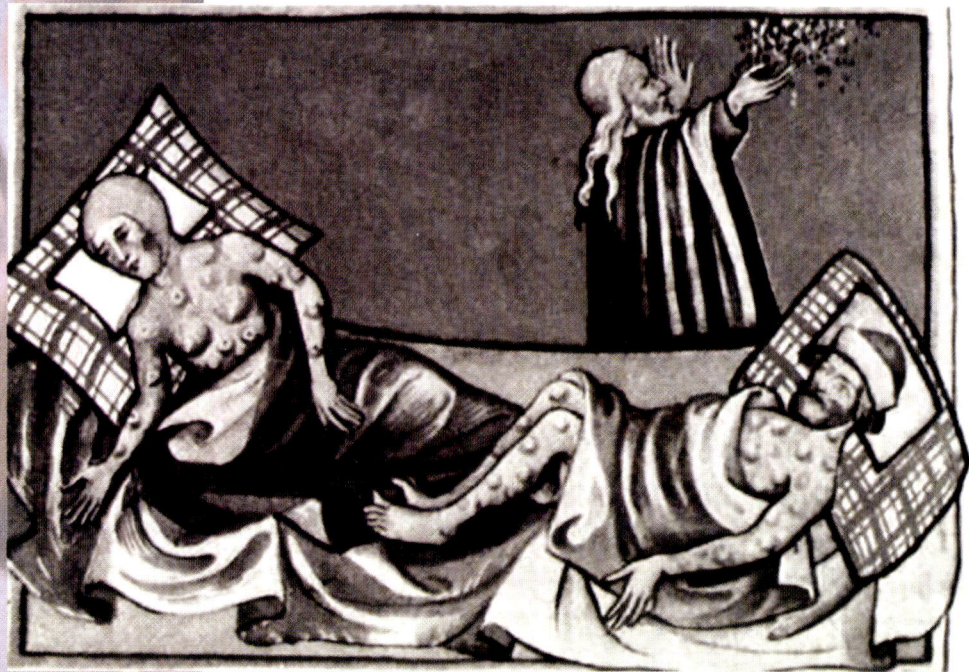

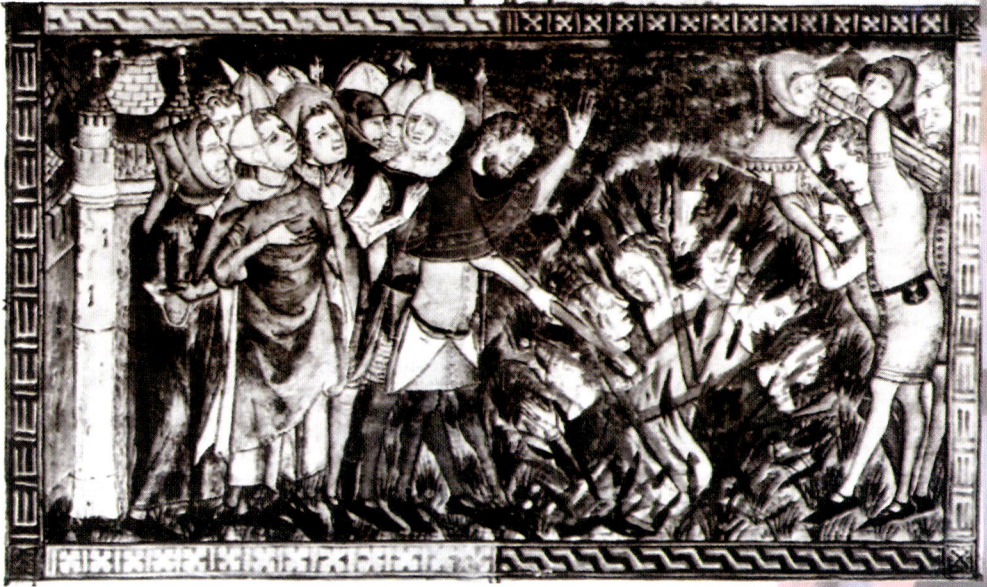

When people are frightened, they sometimes turn on each other, trying to blame the "outsiders" for their problems. During the Middle Ages, Jews were often blamed—and even burned to death—for causing the Plague. Of course the Jews and other groups of people were no more to blame for this epidemic than was anyone else.

gion changed, as they feared that they too would soon die. People did not understand the disease, and they sought someone to take the blame for this terrible affliction. As a result, they began to persecute and kill anyone who looked or acted differently, such as Jews, gypsies, and people with the disease leprosy (which had nothing to do with the Plague). These groups of people did not play any larger role than other people in spreading the disease, and yet they were blamed, simply because they were different.

Political Approaches to Disease

Since governments are supposed to ensure some sort of stability in society, people turn to politicians when there is an outbreak of disease. Often, the government does not fully understand the cause or cure for a disease any more than anyone else does. One of the simplest political approaches to the problem of diseases like the Plague was quarantine, separating infected people from other members of society.

Did You Know?

The Plague spread along trade routes and infected the majority of cities. Scientists today believe that the fleas that lived on rats carried the germ that caused it.

Quarantine has also been used in modern times. During the 1972 outbreak of smallpox in Yugoslavia, for example, the government instituted quarantine and successfully prevented the spread of the disease. In 2007, Andrew Speaker became the first person since 1963 to be placed under U.S. federal quarantine when he flew to Europe knowing that he had tuberculosis and then flew back to the United States, all the while knowing that he had a drug-resistant strain.

Banishment is another method of separating infected people from other members of society. This is similar to

Real People

When foreign traders and sailors arrived on Hawaii's shores, they brought with them a host of diseases the natives there had never known, including leprosy (also called Hansen's disease). Hawaii's ruler, King Kamehameha V, was fearful that this frightening disease would spread throughout his people, and so he quarantined all the lepers in his kingdom and moved them to a settlement colony on the island of Molokai. The Royal Board of Health provided them with supplies and food but no other care.

In 1865, Father Damien, a Dutch missionary, came to the colony, despite the risk to his own life. At the time, 816 lepers were living in the colony. Damien took on the role of doctor as well as priest: he dressed ulcers, built homes and beds, and comforted and taught the people who lived in the colony. He also built coffins and dug graves. Under his leadership, the colony became a functioning community; basic laws were enforced, shacks became painted houses, working farms were organized, and schools were built. Damien died of leprosy at the age of 49.

quarantine, but more permanent; it forces people to leave their homes and be separated from the rest of society if they have a disease. For thousands of years, people who had leprosy were banished from their homes and forced to live in leper colonies. Since people could tell if a person had leprosy by looking at him, lepers were often shunned and treated cruelly. In many cultures, people with leprosy were either encouraged or forced to live (and die) in colonies apart from the rest of society. Until recently, there was no treatment for leprosy; the only way governments knew to control the disease was to separate victims from the rest of the population.

Killing was the most severe form of dealing with infectious diseases. Although it was rarely encouraged by governments, many people let their fear of contracting a disease lead them to commit murder. People are often afraid of things that they do not understand. The practice of killing infected people is related to the widespread persecution of people who look or act differently from the rest of society. Many people with disorders and diseases were killed throughout history because other people did not know enough about the causes and treatment of the conditions.

Even though these methods sometimes helped prevent the spread of a disease, they violated the rights of infected people. According to Article 13 of the United Nation's 1948 Universal Declaration of Human Rights, all people should have the right to move and reside wherever they

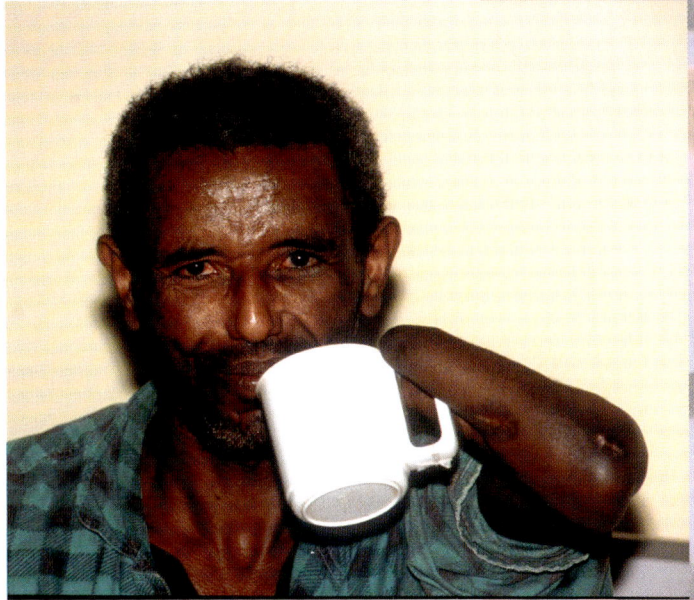

If left untreated, leprosy can cause nerve damage, leading to limb loss and permanent disabilities, such as those shown here. The disease is transmitted via droplets from the nose and mouth, but contrary to the fears of past ages, it is not highly contagious. Today, leprosy is easily treated with a 6–12-month course of multidrug therapy. Despite this, there are still leper colonies in areas where treatment is not widely available or people continue to believe that lepers are "unclean" and should be kept separate from the rest of society.

want within the borders of a state. By forcing certain people to live in designated areas because of a disease, governments were taking away their freedom. Killing infected people also violated their human rights—obviously!—because they were being punished for something that was not their fault. No one wants to have a disease, so it is unfair to treat infected people as less-than-human. And yet too often, even today, society seeks reasons to blame sick people for their illnesses.

As the field of medicine advanced, governments stopped using techniques such as quarantine, killing, and banishment, and instead focused their efforts on funding research. In the late 1930s, for example, scientists developed an effective treatment for leprosy through the medication dapsone. This treatment was further advanced with the development of multidrug therapy in the early 1980s. Many other research breakthroughs came about with the help of government funding. For a while it seemed as though politics might be able to conquer disease forever.

Programs for Public Health

Historically, governments have been very involved in health-related issues. In the 1700s, for instance, the U.S. government recognized the need for health legislation and created a federal network of hospitals for the relief of sick and disabled merchant seamen; this became the earliest foundations of the U.S. Department of Health and Human Services, which came to life formally on May 4, 1980. Most countries have similar programs dedicated to funding and conducting medical research. The Canadian Institutes of Health Research is a major federal agency that aims to create new health knowledge and apply that information in real-world situations. The United Kingdom's Department of Health, India's Ministry of Health and Family Welfare, and China's Ministry of Health all have similar functions.

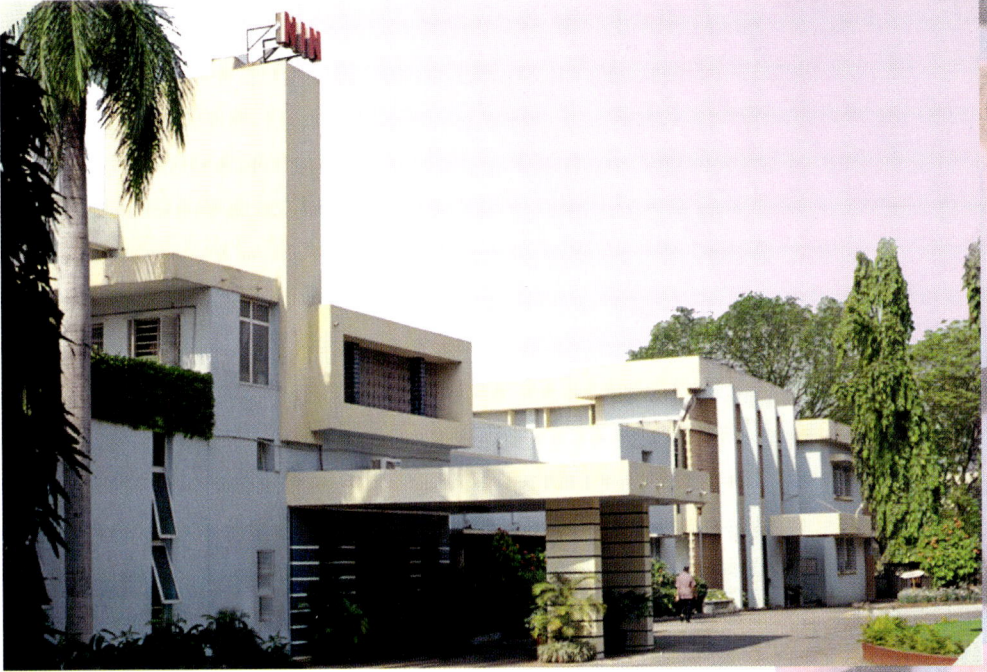

In the United States, the government created the Communicable Disease Center on July 1, 1946. The new agency, which was based on the wartime agency Malaria Control in War Areas, initially engaged 59 percent of its employees in killing mosquitoes to control malaria outbreaks. The agency used its $1 million budget from the government to spray more than six and a half million homes with the insecticide DDT in order to kill mosquitoes, which spread malaria. The CDC eventually expanded its mission to other health issues and changed its name from the Communicable Disease Center to the Centers for Disease Control and Prevention. The agency is now a global leader in dealing with and studying chronic diseases, injury control, environmental health issues, and newer health risks such as the West Nile virus. This and similar organizations in nations around the world demonstrate the greater emphasis on research in dealing with disease.

The Ministry of Health & Family Welfare seeks to protect India's people from AIDS, malaria, leprosy, and malnutrititon.

International Organizations

Health issues affect all people in all parts of the world—but not all countries have the funds, educational programs, or resources necessary for effective research programs that can find the answers to various health problems, including AIDS. What's more, when nations pool their resources, they can often accomplish more. Because of this, nations decided to come together to create international organizations. These bodies also make general guidelines and try to maintain stability on an international scale, which is crucial with the current trends in *globalization*. The United Nations (UN) is the most famous international organization.

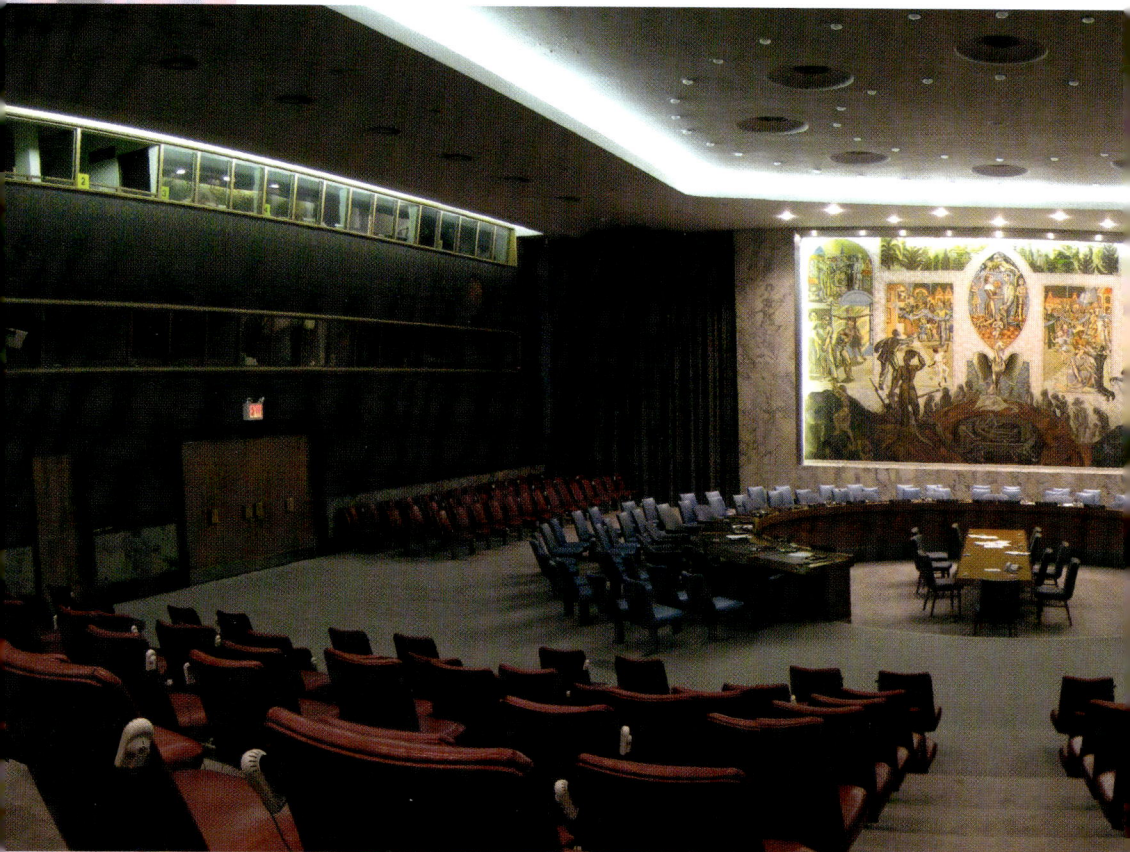

While developing the UN Charter, representatives discussed the need for a global health organization. The World Health Organization, or WHO, was officially established on April 7, 1948. According to its official Web site, the core functions of the WHO are:

- providing leadership on health matters and shaping partnerships where joint action is needed.
- deciding on a research plan and encouraging the spread of knowledge between nations.
- setting standards for all nations and making sure that they're followed.
- shaping policies based on both facts and morals.

The United Nations provides a meeting place where the world's leaders can come together to discuss problems such as AIDS—and seek to join forces to find solutions.

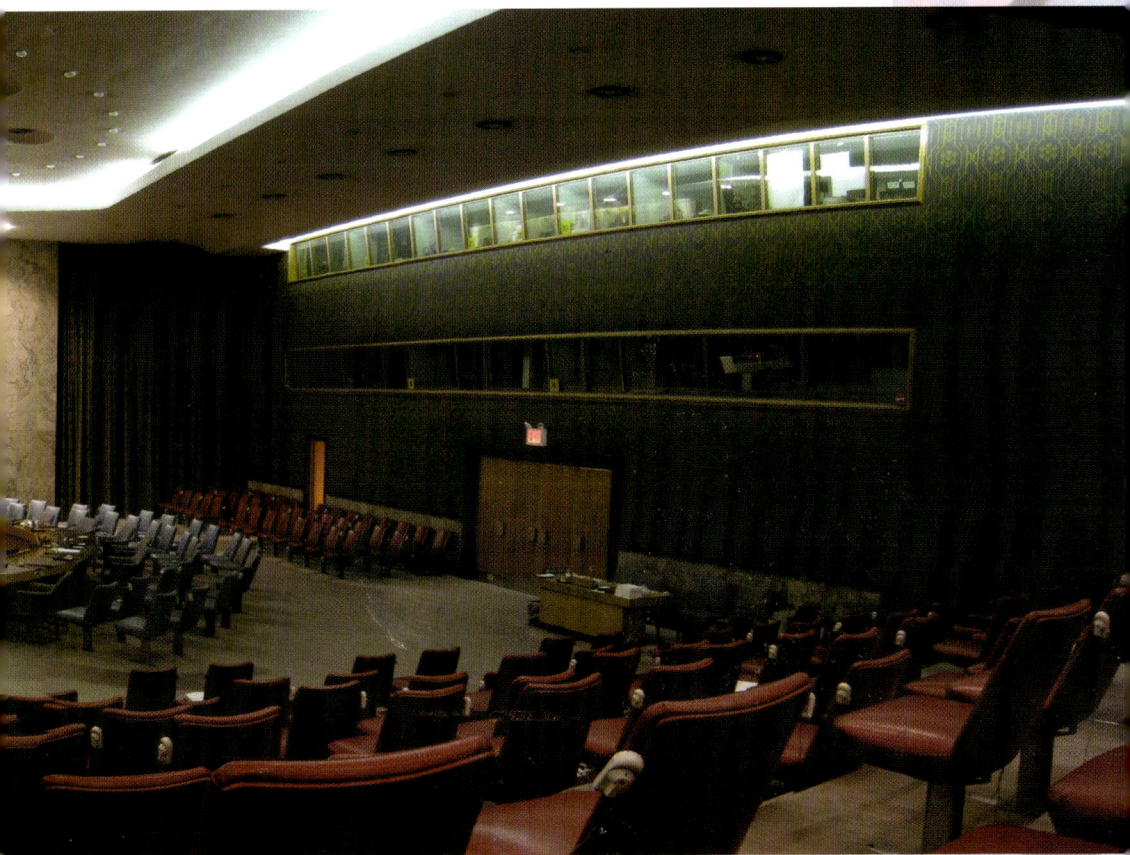

- providing technical support, encouraging change, and building institutions capable of sustaining themselves.
- keeping watch on the world's health situation and health trends.

Since its creation, the WHO has provided millions of dollars in medical supplies to developing nations and areas affected by natural disasters. The STEPS surveillance program allows countries to monitor health trends—such as the number of people infected with a disease—with the help of the WHO. By gathering information and assessing health needs in countries, the WHO can distribute aid accordingly. Using funds from voluntary contributions and contributions from member states of the UN, the WHO spends the majority of its budget on health interventions, such as reducing maternal and child *mortality* and responding to epidemics. The remainder of the budget is spent improving the quality of medicines and technologies, supporting member states, and researching the factors that contribute to health. Over the years, the UN and WHO have helped improve global health.

Vaccinations

The World Health Organisation's symbol; the WHO's constitution states that its objective "is the attainment by all peoples of the highest possible level of health," with its major task being to combat disease and to promote the general health of the people of the world.

One of the most effective means of improving global health is through vaccinations. A vaccination is a means of producing immunity to a disease by exposing a person to a weakened form of the germ that causes the disease. Before vaccinations

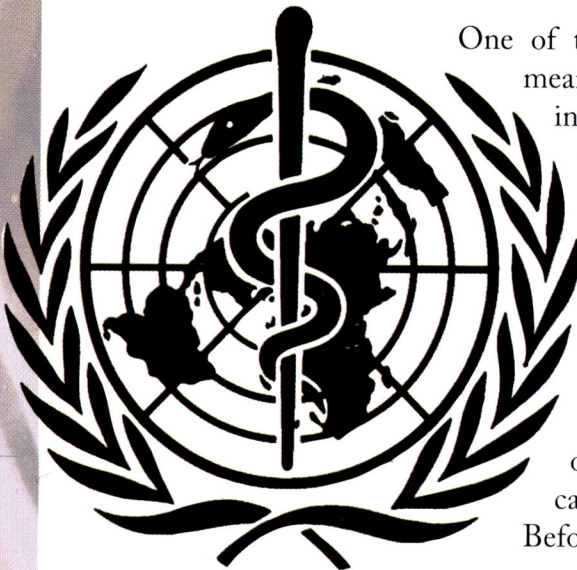

were developed, many people died of diseases such as smallpox and measles.

In 1796, Edward Jenner observed that many milkmaids who caught the cowpox virus did not catch smallpox, so he created a vaccine based on these findings. The result was the first successful vaccine ever to be developed. On May 8, 1980, the Thirty-Third World Health Assembly declared that the WHO had essentially eliminated smallpox through an intense worldwide search and vaccination program. Although there have been incidents of smallpox since then, people can be saved if they are vaccinated within four days of exposure to the virus.

Other vaccines have also been effective. In 1955, Dr. Jonas Salk developed the first vaccine against polio. This development lessened the fear that people had of a disease that had afflicted many people throughout history, including U.S. President Franklin D. Roosevelt. The WHO and

Did You Know?

Smallpox is estimated to have killed 400,000 Europeans every year in the eighteenth century. Between 20 and 60 percent of all people infected with smallpox died from the disease.

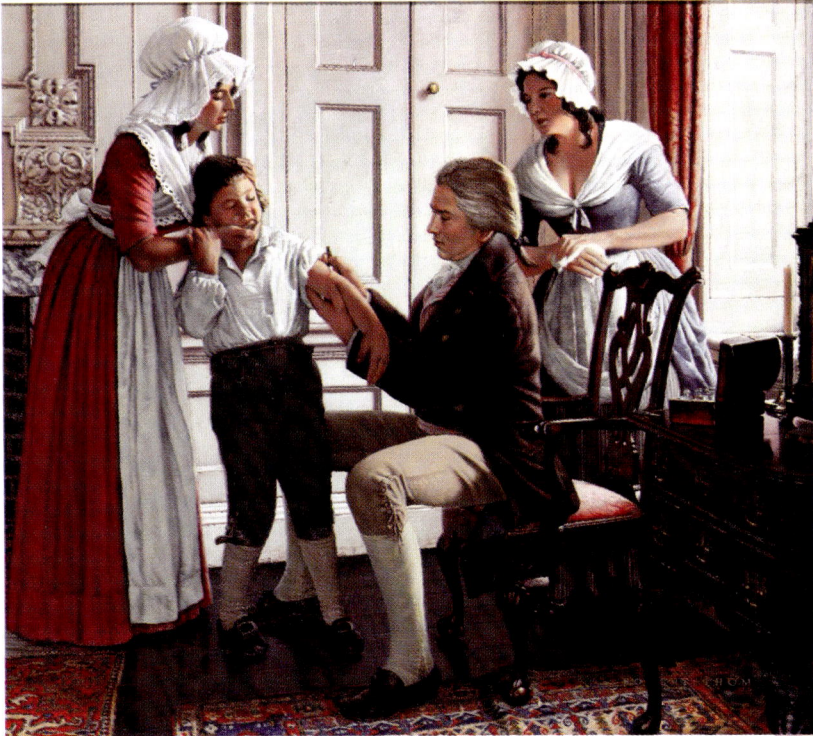

This painting depicts the use of the first Western vaccine: the cowpox vaccine to protect against smallpox. Edward Jenner, a rural English doctor, is shown injecting his first patient, James Phipps, in 1796, using fluid obtained from scratches on the hand of dairymaid Sarah Nelmes, standing behind him.

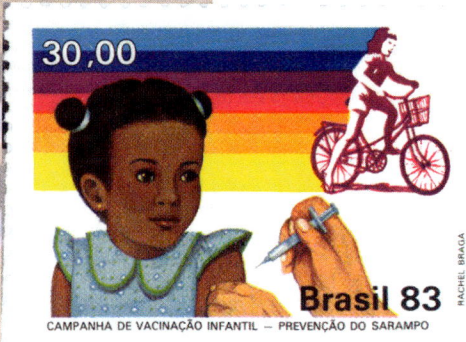

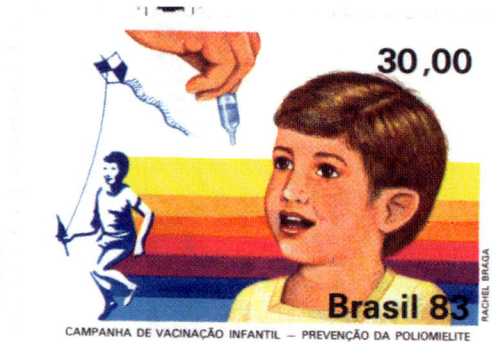

These postage stamps demonstrate the Brazilian government's efforts to fight measles and polio through vaccinations.

Did You Know?

Records show that the first vaccines were used by the Chinese as early as 200 BCE.

other organizations used the vaccine to lower the number of polio-endemic countries from more than 125 in 1988 to only four (India, Afghanistan, Nigeria, and Pakistan) in 2008. The measles vaccine was licensed in the U.S. in 1963. Children in many of the developed nations are usually given the combination measles, mumps, and rubella vaccine at the age of one year, and they are given a booster shot before they can enter school. Despite the success of this vaccine in developed nations, measles remains one of the leading causes of death among young children in

An American postage stamp promotes government-funded health research.

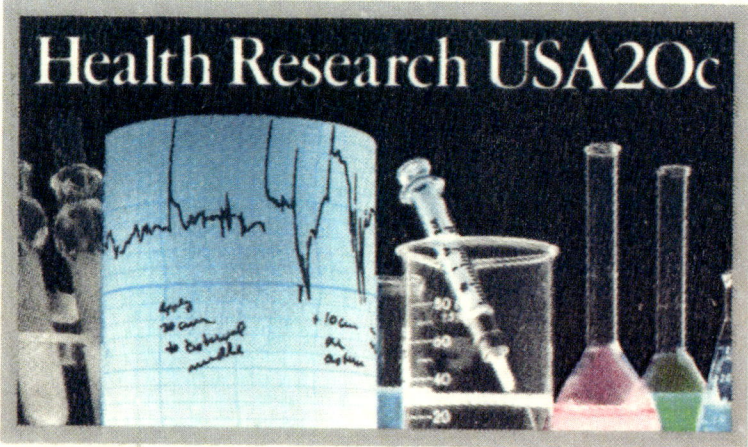

developing nations. With the development of vaccines and new medical breakthroughs, organizations such as the WHO continue to face the challenge of administering vaccines to poor countries.

Governments and AIDS

The WHO and other government-sponsored organizations are excellent examples of politics working on behalf of those who are sick, including those with AIDS. Unfortunately, however, not everyone agrees on how much money should be spent on solving the enormous problem AIDS poses to the world. Controversies like this mean that politicians spend more time vying for power and less time finding solutions.

When it comes to a disease like AIDS, the modern-day version of the Plague, emotions run high. People feel strongly on both sides of many AIDS issues, and their opinions shape the politicians who run our world. This has been the case ever since AIDS was first recognized back in the 1970s—and the controversies have continued into the twenty-first century.

Ask the Doctor

Q: I heard that there is a vaccine for cancer. Is this true?

Not for all types of cancer. You probably heard of the cervical cancer vaccine, known as Gardasil. This is a very significant breakthrough, since about 10,000 women in the U.S. are diagnosed with cervical cancer every year, and 4,000 die from it. The WHO estimated that there were 500,000 new cases of cervical cancer worldwide in 2005. The reason why there is a vaccine for cervical cancer and not for other kinds of cancer is because researchers discovered that cervical cancer is caused by the human papillomavirus (HPV). Since HPV spreads through sexual contact, many doctors recommend that the girls get the vaccine between ages 11 and 12, before they are likely to encounter the virus. As with any vaccine, people have health concerns and everyone should ask her doctor before deciding to get the series of three injections. Cancer is a very complicated illness, and researchers are still trying to find a cure for other types.

STRAIGHT FROM THE SOURCE

Plague's Eyewitness Account

(From the fourteenth-century account of Agnolo di Tura of Siena, Italy.)

The mortality in Siena began in May. It was a cruel and horrible thing. . . . It seemed that almost everyone became stupefied seeing the pain. It is impossible for the human tongue to recount the awful truth. Indeed, one who did not see such horribleness can be called blessed. The victims died almost immediately. They would swell beneath the armpits and in the groin, and fall over while talking. Father abandoned child, wife husband, one brother another; for this illness seemed to strike through breath and sight. And so they died. None could be found to bury the dead for money or friendship. Members of a household brought their dead to a ditch as best they could, without priest, without divine offices. In many places in Siena great pits were dug and piled deep with the multitude of dead. And they died by the hundreds, both day and night, and all were thrown in those ditches and covered with earth. And as soon as those ditches were filled, more were dug. I, Agnolo di Tura . . . buried my five children with my own hands. . . . And so many died that all believed it was the end of the world.

What Do You Think?

- Why do you think no one could be found to bury the dead "for money or friendship"?

- In what ways do you think people's reactions to AIDS is similar to what Agnolo di Tura describes here?

- How was the Plague worse than AIDS?

Find Out More

To find out more about historical and current means of dealing with diseases, check out these Web sites:

Diseases in History

www.bignell.uk.com/disease_in_history.htm

The History of Diseases

www.mla-hhss.org/histdis.htm

Here's what you need to know

- Since gay men were the first people to be diagnosed with AIDS, many people ignored the disease and treated AIDS patients with the same discrimination they treated homosexuals.

- People were initially reluctant to discuss HIV/AIDS because they felt uncomfortable talking about sex and drug use.

- Liberals pushed for condom distribution and needle exchange programs, but conservatives thought that these programs would encourage premarital sex and drug use.

- HIV/AIDS patients continue to face discrimination because people do not understand the disease and are afraid that they might somehow contract HIV from them.

Words to Understand

A *taboo* is something that society considers unacceptable or improper.

Conservative means traditional or wanting to preserve existing or past conditions.

To be *polarized* means that society is broken into opposing groups with opposite attitudes.

Liberal means favoring progress or reform and encouraging individual freedom.

Abstinence is the practice of not having sex. Abstinence-only education teaches students why they should not have sex but does not teach them how to have sex safely.

Transgender refers to people who identify with the opposite sex, such as a person who was born a man but feels truly like a woman.

An *advocate* is someone who supports or promotes a cause, such as the rights of gays and lesbians.

4

AIDS and Political Controversies

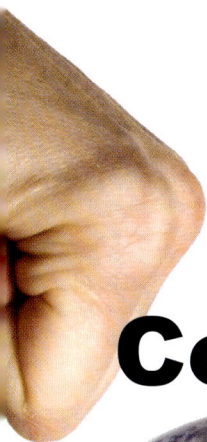

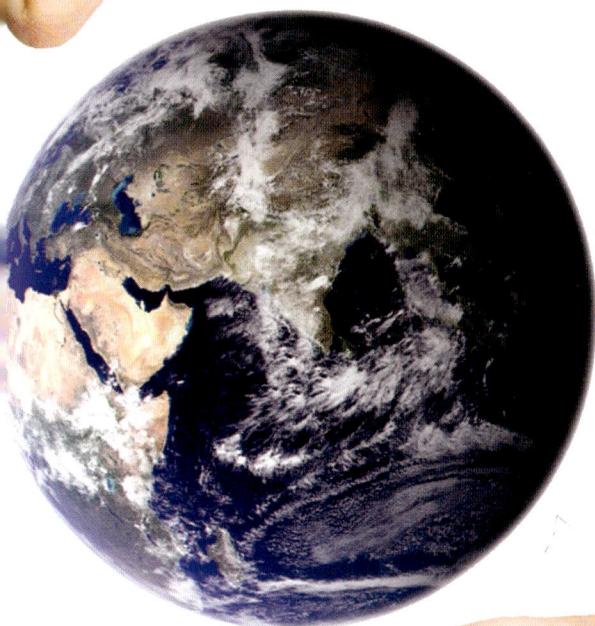

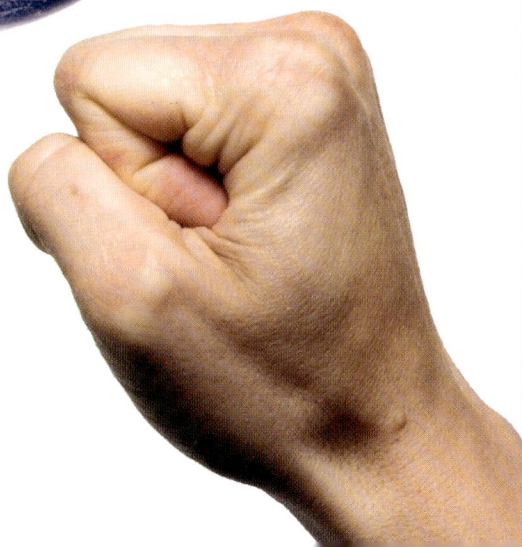

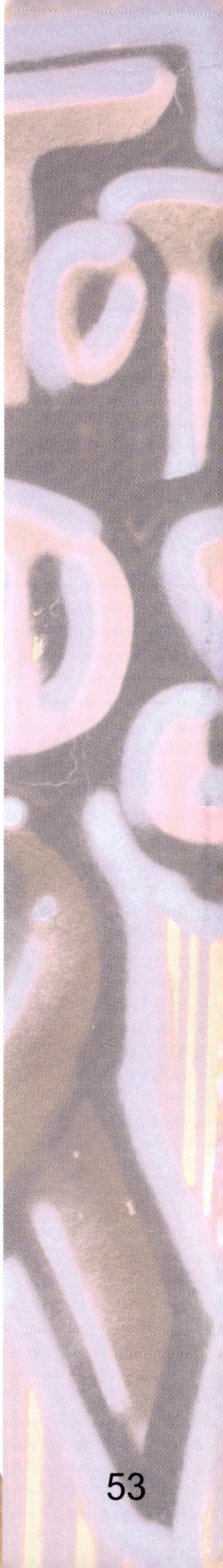

As you've probably noticed, people often disagree when it comes to political issues. This is why people who otherwise get along well might become upset if they begin a political discussion. In a democratic system, such as Australia, the United Kingdom, or the United States, for example, people can voice their beliefs through voting for candidates or parties who have similar ideas to their own. Of course, everyone has the right to his or her own opinion, and various factors influence how people think. But because different groups of people have different ideas about AIDS, political controversies have raged over this disease.

Ever since AIDS was identified back in the 1980s, many people thought the disease was different from other major illnesses because it can be passed through sexual intercourse. In fact, this is not the only way that people can contract HIV, but it was the first means of transmission

AIDS was initially associated nearly exclusively with homosexuals—which meant it created political controversies right from the beginning, since many people were uncomfortable or uncertain about their beliefs in regards to homosexuality. AIDS meant that people had to confront this issue.

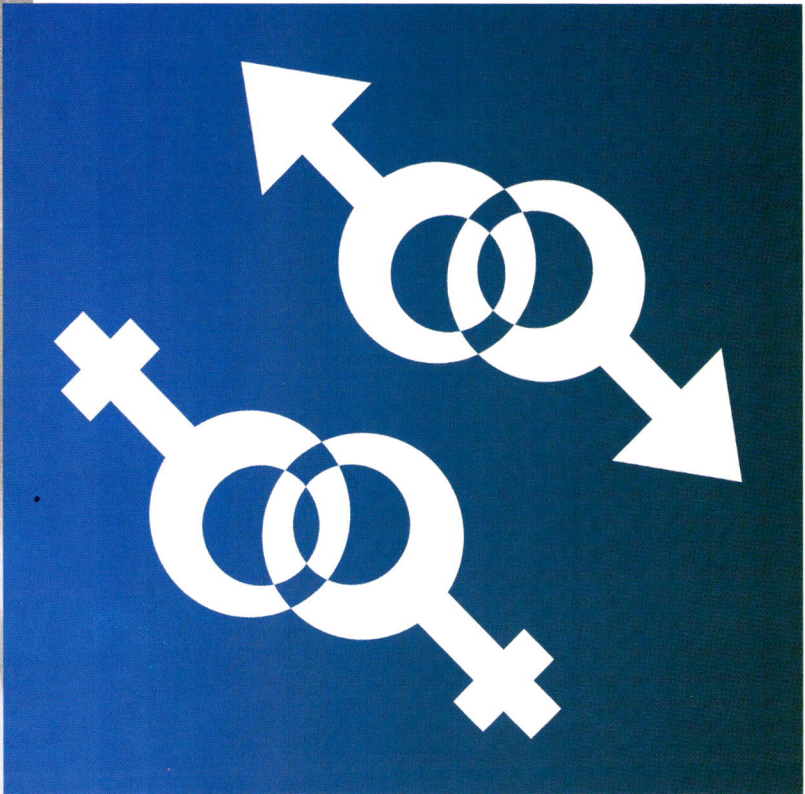

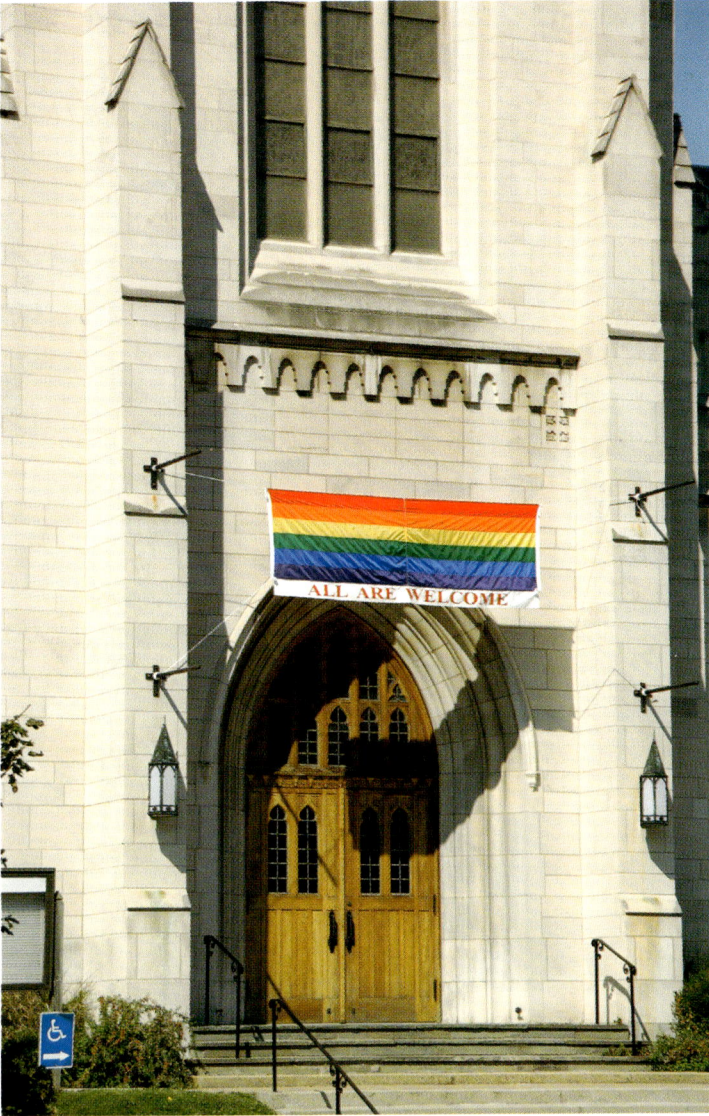

Not all religious groups took a stand against homosexuality. This church proclaimed its acceptance of homosexuals with its rainbow banner.

ALL ARE WELCOME

Did You Know?

Researchers began to notice the disease that would later be called AIDS when at least eight young gay men in New York were diagnosed with an aggressive form of the rare cancer Kaposi's Sarcoma in early 1981. There was also an increase in the rare lung infection Pneumocystis carinii pneumonia in New York and California.

that the general population heard about when researchers began to study the disease. At first, people were reluctant to discuss the disease because sex is a social *taboo*; people aren't supposed to talk about it openly. People's attitudes about HIV/AIDS were (and often still are) tied to their attitudes about sex and alternative lifestyles. Although these attitudes impacted political decisions in many Western nations in North America and Europe, they have had an even greater influence in more **conservative** countries, where people never talk about sex or homosexuality.

Identifying AIDS

It's difficult today to imagine a world without AIDS. However, just a few decades ago, no one had heard of the disease. When AIDS was first recognized in 1981, the first AIDS patients were mainly homosexual American men.

Many people were uncomfortable with the idea of homosexuality. Some religious groups taught that homosexuality was a sin, and most people simply did not understand or know anyone who fell into this category. Homosexuals were generally considered to be "abnormal" or "perverted"; in other words, they were thought to be weird sex maniacs. Members of the homosexual community were often discriminated against, and many times

Antibodies are a part of your body's defense system. The presence of HIV triggers your body to make a certain kind of antibody to protect itself; doctors use the presence of this antibody as a way to tell if a person has the virus.

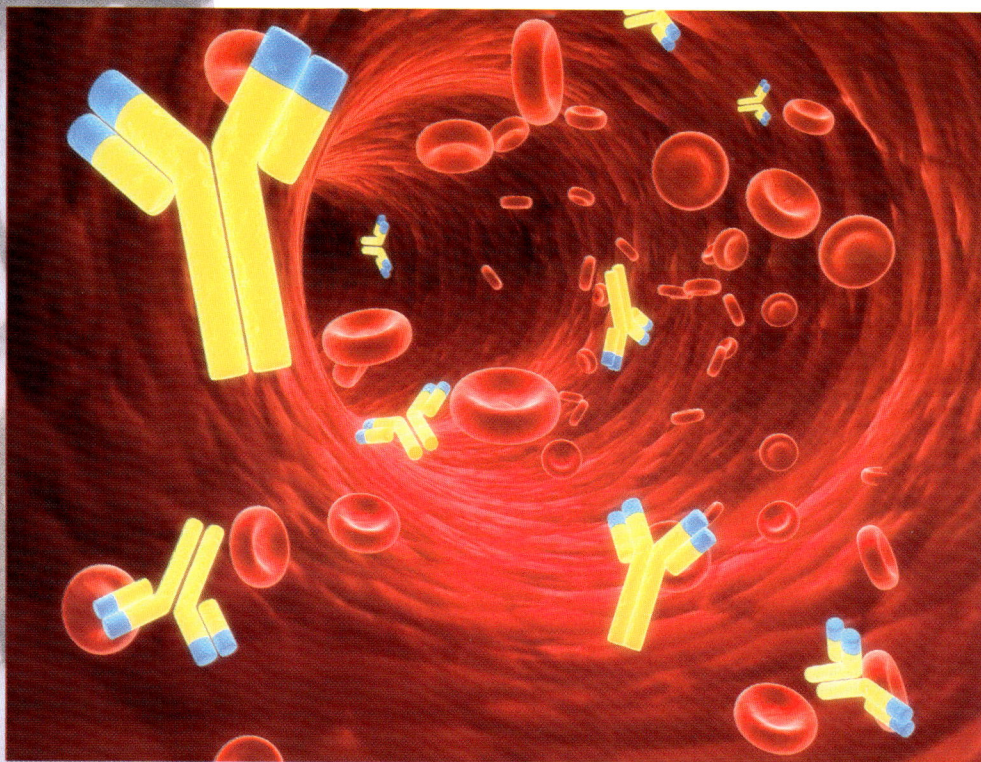

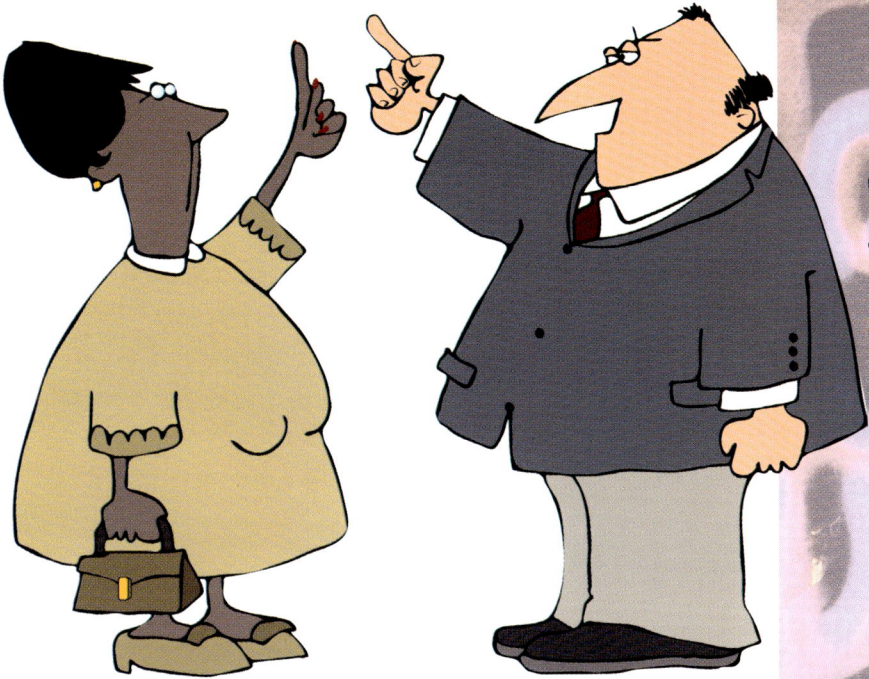

People are bound to disagree. However, when groups of people within a single country look at the world in very different ways, it often leads from individual arguments to bigger political controversies.

they were attacked or killed. Because they did not want to face persecution, many people were afraid to admit that they were homosexual. As a result, communities acted as though homosexuality did not exist. AIDS changed all that.

When reports of AIDS became publicized, people had to face that homosexuality was real. This made many conservative communities uncomfortable, and some people refused to recognize AIDS, just as they had refused to recognize homosexuality as a lifestyle. Researchers and doctors were still trying to learn more about the new disease, and the lack of information made people speculate about the causes and reasons for AIDS. Some people labeled it a "gay disease" and thought that they were safe because the disease wasn't *their* problem. Religious leaders even expressed the belief that AIDS was a punishment from God for the sinfulness of homosexual lifestyles.

As mainstream society either ignored or persecuted homosexuals, researchers were at work trying to under-

Did You Know?

The FDA is an agency within the U.S. Department of Health and Human Services, and its responsibilities include ensuring that new drugs and medications are safe for use by the public.

stand AIDS. In 1982, the U.S. Food and Drug Administration, a government organization known as the FDA, received the first submission for the treatment of AIDS. In this way, the American government contributed to initial information and discoveries about AIDS.

In 1984, researchers identified a human retrovirus, the Human Immunodeficiency Virus (HIV), as the cause of AIDS. The following year, the FDA approved the first enzyme-linked immunosorbant assay (ELISA) test kit to screen for antibodies to HIV. This allowed doctors for the first time to test for HIV, but it was replaced by a better blood test in 1987. Also in 1987, the FDA approved AZT, which was the first drug approved for the treatment of AIDS. In just a few years since the discovery of AIDS,

Marchers in a parade in Toronto, Canada, show their solidarity with the gay community's fight against AIDS.

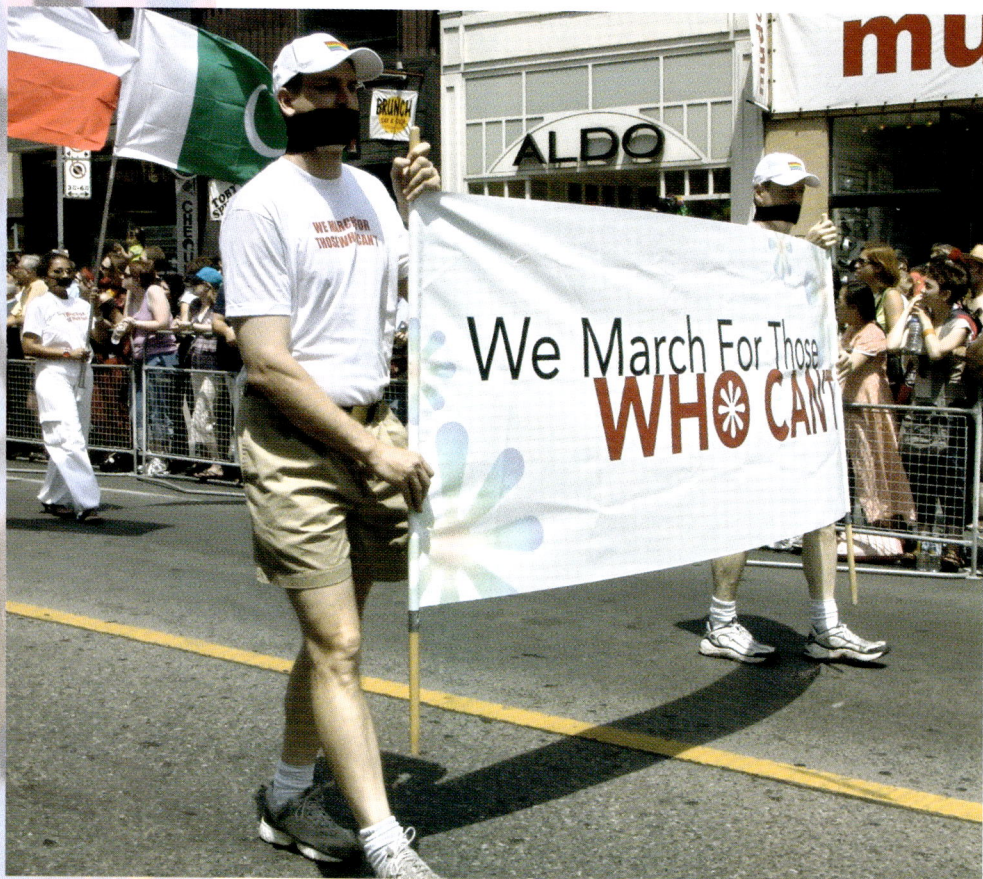

steps were made to find effective treatment for the disease, and the American government played an important role in this process.

Many people, however, believed that not enough progress was being made fast enough. If this disease had been first identified in the children of rich white people, for instance, wouldn't the government have done more to find the answers that would put an end to the disease? Researchers were learning more about the disease, but most people still did not understand the significance of these findings, and many people still thought that only gay men could have AIDS. Unfortunately, this was a group of people that not everyone cared all that much about.

Liberal and Conservative Politics

As more cases of HIV/AIDS were reported and more scientific breakthroughs were made, society became *polarized*. The two main attitudes about HIV/AIDS were based on the major political groups within the United States: liberals and conservatives. *Liberals* typically want the government to take care of all citizens and are accepting of alternative lifestyles, such as homosexuality; they are less likely to say that a person is making a "wrong" decision, because they are open to many possibilities and believe that people can act or think however they personally see fit. Conservatives, meanwhile, are people who tend to avoid discussing homosexuality or sexual intercourse in general, because those topics have traditionally been social taboos. Conservatives often have religious affiliations. Clearly, liberals and conservatives disagree on many issues. AIDS was no different.

Historically, premarital sex—sex between people who were not married—was frowned upon in the United States. Adults sometimes pretended that teenagers were not having sex despite rising numbers of unwed teen mothers. Religion plays a large role in shaping beliefs and attitudes, and many religions condemn premarital sex. Traditionally, sex education in schools only told students

Did You Know?

Many people are conservative on some issues and liberal on others. Moderates fall somewhere in between the two groups. Neither group is superior, and they both have made good decisions, as well as bad ones.

that they should maintain a policy of **abstinence**; many adults feared that telling students how to have safer sex and giving them information about condoms and other forms of contraception would encourage more teenagers to have sex. Instead of giving students information, educators hoped that keeping them in the dark would discourage them from having sex. This is a mainly conservative position. Liberals usually believe that students should be given information about contraceptives and ways of protecting themselves from pregnancy and STIs. They reason that teenagers will have sex either way, so they might as well know how to go about it safely. In the past few decades, this abstinence-only versus comprehensive sex education debate has divided many school districts. Meanwhile, however, homosexual sex was left out of the discussion altogether.

Another difference between liberals and conservatives is their level of acceptance of alternative sexual identities—people who do not identify with the heterosexual lifestyle and instead consider themselves lesbian, gay, bisexual, **transgender**, or another identity. Traditionally, society has discriminated against people with alternative lifestyles. They were often seen as sinful, unhealthy, or abnormal. This view is more common among conservatives, although certainly not all conservatives have this opinion. In general, conservatives are less likely to talk about alternative lifestyles. Liberals are often more open **advocates** for gay rights and push for laws against discrimination.

Beliefs about sexuality, about what is right and wrong, and about how God wants people to live are often very deeply felt. Conservatives and liberals both felt that these were deeply moral questions. A common ground to talk about viewpoints on these issues was difficult to find.

Condom Distribution

It's no surprise that people disagreed about how to deal with HIV/AIDS. Since many people initially considered the disease a problem only for homosexuals, conservatives

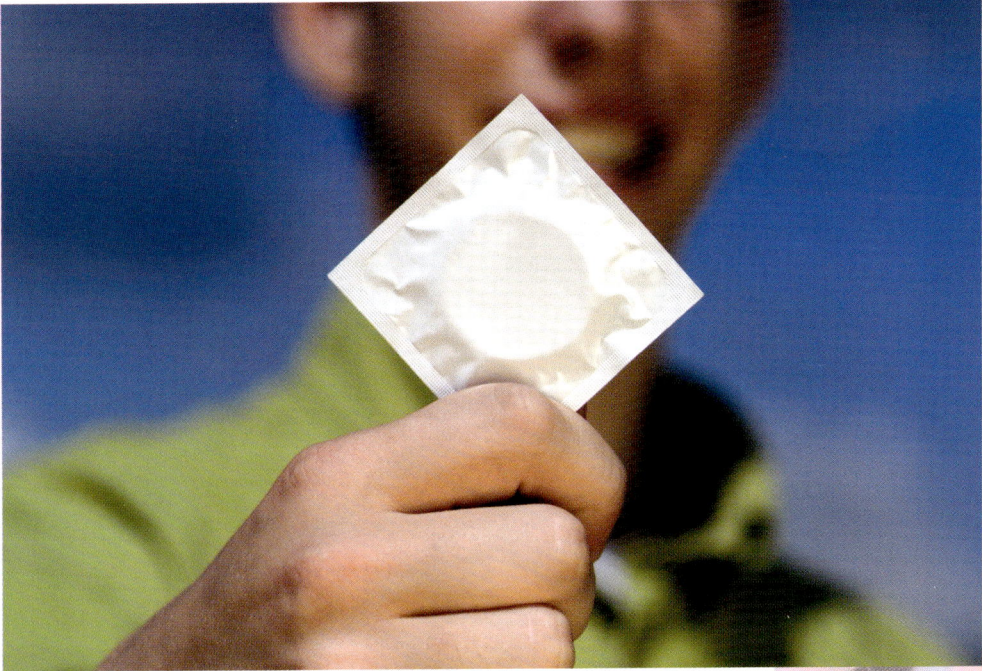

were reluctant to address the issue at all. The identification of HIV/AIDS as a significant issue in society made many people favor a comprehensive sex education program so that students would know how to properly use condoms and protect themselves from the disease. Some liberals suggested that schools distribute condoms to students, whereas many conservatives again thought that such methods would encourage students to have sex.

Needle-Exchange Programs

Another controversial issue involved needle-exchange programs. Since HIV can be spread through the bloodstream, people who use intravenous drugs are at a high risk of contracting HIV if they use the same needles as other drug users. Often, these drugs, such as heroin, are among the most addictive, and drug users have an extremely difficult time quitting even if they want to. As a result, some people are in favor of a needle-exchange program, where drug users can go to a specific location to turn in their

Distributing condoms to teenagers is a very controversial issue. Those who are for it say that it is better to encourage adolescents to practice safer sex, while those who argue against it insist that the best approach is to teach abstinence to teens.

Real People

When Jeremiah Johnson was volunteering with the government volunteer service the Peace Corps, he thought that he was helping make a difference in the world. He was stationed in Ukraine, and he felt that he was helping a lot of people there.

Then, in January 2008, Jeremiah had a scheduled medical examination in Kiev, the capitol of Ukraine. When the doctor told him that he was HIV-positive, he knew that the plans he had for the future would be changed. Ukrainian law does not permit anyone with HIV to volunteer in the country. In fact, any foreigner working in Ukraine with a visa lasting more than three months is required to undergo HIV tests. A few days after Jeremiah received the test results, the Peace Corps' country director for Ukraine told Jeremiah to return to Washington, D.C.

Back in the U.S., Jeremiah had to have another medical exam in February. He was given a "medical separation" from the Peace Corps, and the separation notice said that his medical condition would take longer than 45 days to resolve itself and that he would be "medically unable to perform [his] volunteer assignment." The Peace Corps did not try to help him find another country where he could volunteer; they simply told him that he could no longer serve with them.

Devastated, Jeremiah realized that he was being discriminated against. People with HIV are not necessarily unable to perform duties, and if they are aware of their condition they can take extra precautions to avoid infecting other people. With the help of the ACLU, Jeremiah hopes to make sure the Peace Corps and other government organizations follow federal antidiscrimination laws.

used needles and receive clean needles. This is controversial, because other people believe it would encourage drug use. The arguments for and against this program are similar to those involving condom distribution in schools: the advocates say that people are going to do drugs either way, so they might as well be protected from HIV, while those who are against this policy insist that by helping drug users protect themselves from HIV, such a program would condone drug use.

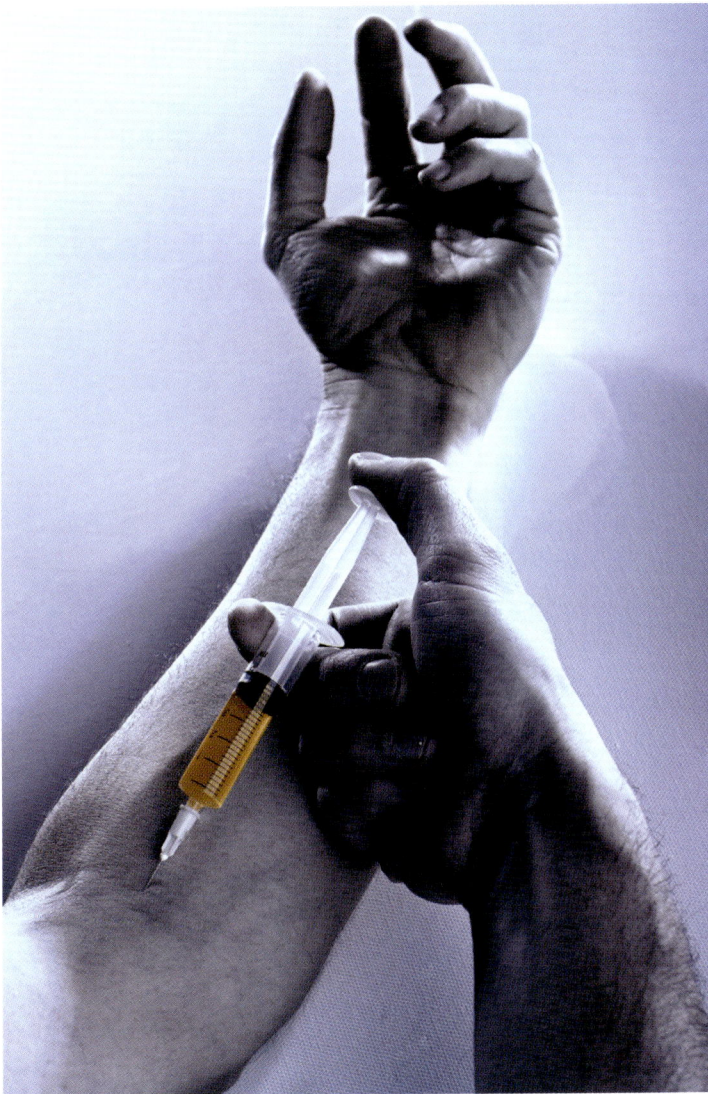

In many nations, heroin use is illegal. Does this mean that distributing clean needles to drug users encourages crime? Or does distributing clean needles merely prevent the spread of HIV? What do you think?

Gender Issues

As other parts of the world besides America began to recognize the AIDS crisis, new political issues came to light. In many African nations, for example, gender issues of control and power within heterosexual relationships played an important role in HIV transmission. Men often have greater sexual freedom than women, and economic pressures often mean that men travel to find work. In a culture where it is accepted behavior for men to seek out prostitutes, this means that these men often bring HIV back home with them to their wives, who have no means to protect themselves. Liberal politicians in these regions believe that the empowerment of women is an essential step in any HIV/AIDS prevention program—while more conservative and traditional politicians have resisted such efforts.

Because AIDS is transmitted sexually, its issues touch on many other complicated and deeply felt beliefs, including how women are viewed within a society. Some people believe that women must be empowered so that they can protect themselves against AIDS (and abuse); meanwhile, people on the other side of the issue believe that traditional beliefs, including those about the roles of men and women, must be respected. This issue is especially relevant to HIV transmission in many African countries.

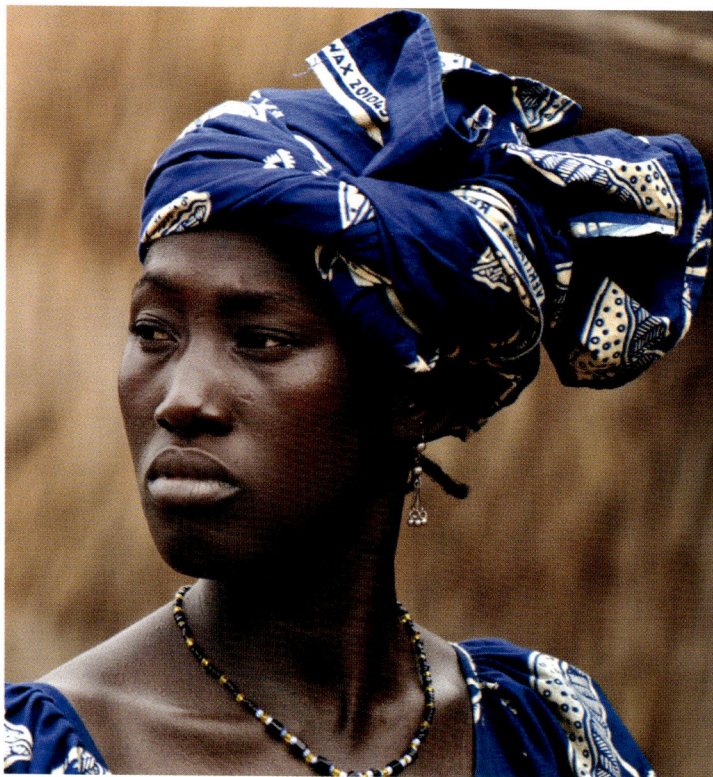

Discrimination

Discrimination is another issue that has brought controversy to AIDS politics. Around the world, many nations believe that all people are entitled to certain human rights and equal treatment. Politicians are often held responsible for ensuring that people do not face discrimination. However, because many people did not fully understand how AIDS was transmitted, they feared they would get the disease just by touching or being near an HIV-positive person. This misinformation made employers reluctant to hire people with the disease; it made schools refuse to let HIV-positive children attend classes; and it made people afraid to work, play, or worship with those who had the virus.

Organizations such as the American Civil Liberties Union stepped into the controversy and insisted that anti-discrimination laws be upheld. If an employer were to fire someone only on the basis that he was HIV-positive, for example, the ACLU would represent the HIV-positive person in a lawsuit because that person did not receive equal, fair treatment. Despite laws to prevent discrimination against people based on their medical status, prejudice still existed.

Unfortunately, that prejudice still exists today—and it continues to shape the world's politics.

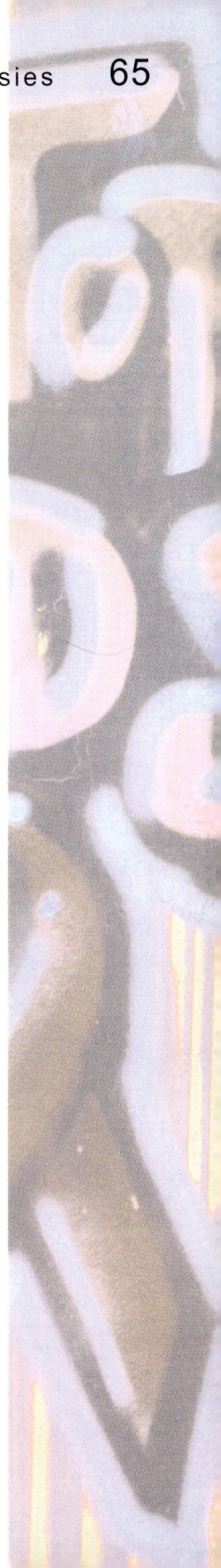

STRAIGHT FROM THE SOURCE

(From Nora Volkow, Director, U.S. National Institute on Drug Abuse, Aug. 4, 2004)

While it is not feasible to do a randomized controlled trial of the effectiveness of needle or syringe exchange programs (NEPs/SEPs) in reducing HIV incidence, the majority of studies have shown that NEPs/SEPs are strongly associated with reductions in the spread of HIV when used as a component of comprehensive approach to HIV prevention. NEPs/SEPs increase the availability of sterile syringes and other injection equipment, and for exchange participants, this decreases the fraction of needles in circulation that are contaminated. This lower fraction of contaminated needles reduces the risk of injection with a contaminated needle and lowers the risk of HIV transmission.

In addition to decreasing HIV infected needles in circulation through the physical exchange of syringes, most NEPs/SEPs are part of a comprehensive HIV prevention effort that may include education on risk reduction, and referral to drug addiction treatment, job or other social services, and these interventions may be responsible for a significant part of the overall effectiveness of NEPs/SEPs. NEPs/SEPs also provide an opportunity to reach out to populations that are often difficult to engage in treatment."

What Do You Think?

- Why is the author, Nora Volkow, a supporter of needle- and syringe-exchange programs?

- Are there any other arguments for these programs that were not mentioned in this document?

- What might someone from the opposing side say in response to this document?

- Do you think that these programs encourage people to do drugs?

- If it were up to you, how would you solve this dilemma?

Find Out More

To learn more about HIV and controversies surrounding it, check out these Web sites:

Food and Drug Administration Website HIV/AIDS Timeline
www.fda.gov/oashi/aids/miles.html

Voices of Youth: HIV and AIDS
www.unicef.org/voy/explore/aids/explore_aids.php

For information about needle exchange programs and HIV, see:
www.drugwarfacts.org

Here's what you need to know

- Developing countries do not have the money to fund medical research or to institute educational programs about HIV/AIDS.
- Different literacy rates around the world make it difficult to teach people about HIV/AIDS.
- Some people see international intervention as outsiders imposing their culture on other peoples.
- The most effective treatment for HIV involves a variety of medications.
- Most people in developing countries who need HIV/AIDS treatments in order to survive do not have access to those medications, despite global efforts.
- Medical research raises many ethical and financial debates.

Words to Understand

Stigma is the condition of being viewed by society with disapproval because of a particular attribute or characteristic.

A *humanitarian* is someone who promotes the welfare of human beings.

Antiretroviral drugs are medicines that fight retroviruses, such as HIV.

Highly Active Antiretroviral Therapy refers to a combination of three or more antiretroviral drugs used to treat HIV. It is often used to prolong the onset of AIDS.

A *placebo* is a substance that has no medical effects but is given to patients to serve as a control, or means of comparison, in medical research.

5
Modern-Day Issues

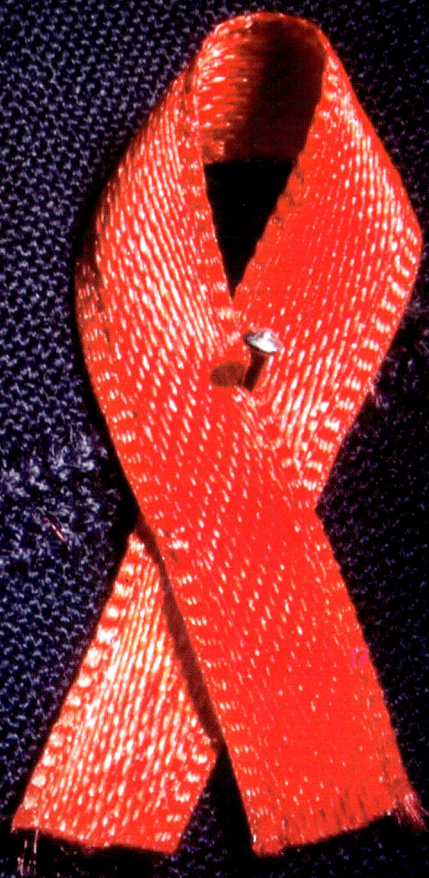

Did You Know?

The literacy rate, which is usually defined as the percentage of the population over age 15 that can read, is 99% in the United States, but only 82% in the whole world. In the African country of Burkina Faso, the literacy rate is only 21.8%.

Even though researchers and societies have come a long way since the first cases of AIDS were reported, we still face challenges related to the disease. Doctors now know how to diagnose HIV/AIDS, how to prevent other people from being infected, and how to treat HIV patients using a variety of medicines. Also, more people are learning about the disease and becoming more involved in helping end discrimination against HIV-positive people. In many communities, the *stigma* of being HIV-positive is being replaced with compassion and support. As education programs are expanded and more research is funded, it looks as though our world is moving closer every day to eliminating AIDS.

However, that goal is still difficult to achieve. Each day, more people are infected with HIV and more people die from AIDS around the world. The education and research programs are making important progress, but they continue to face roadblocks from people who do not fully understand HIV/AIDS and governments who resist these prevention methods. Despite the fact that many people have developed a greater understanding of the disease, HIV/AIDS patients are still treated unfairly in many communities. When politics gets involved, the situation can become very complicated.

Dealing with AIDS Across Borders

One of the most difficult challenges to the fight against HIV/AIDS is global inequalities. Although researchers in developed nations have the time and resources to study the disease, many governments can hardly manage to ensure that all their citizens have enough food and water to survive; there are simply no resources for funding research programs that require expensive medical technologies. In these situations, developing countries must rely on international organizations, such as the UN, and *humanitarian* groups.

Education is one of the most important weapons in the fight against AIDS—but like everything, it costs money.

Most international organizations rely on donations from member countries, and politicians in those nations usually try to direct their money to domestic issues before they will donate to campaigns in other countries. If the wealthiest nations do not support HIV/AIDS education around the world, no progress will be made in this area.

Education becomes even more difficult in countries where large segments of the populations can't read or write. How can people learn how to protect themselves from HIV/AIDS if they cannot read newspapers or pamphlets, and they have no access to television or radio? In developed nations, most people learn about safer sex and AIDS prevention while they are in school—but people in developing countries often do not have access to sex education classes. Schools offer a pipeline for AIDS edu-

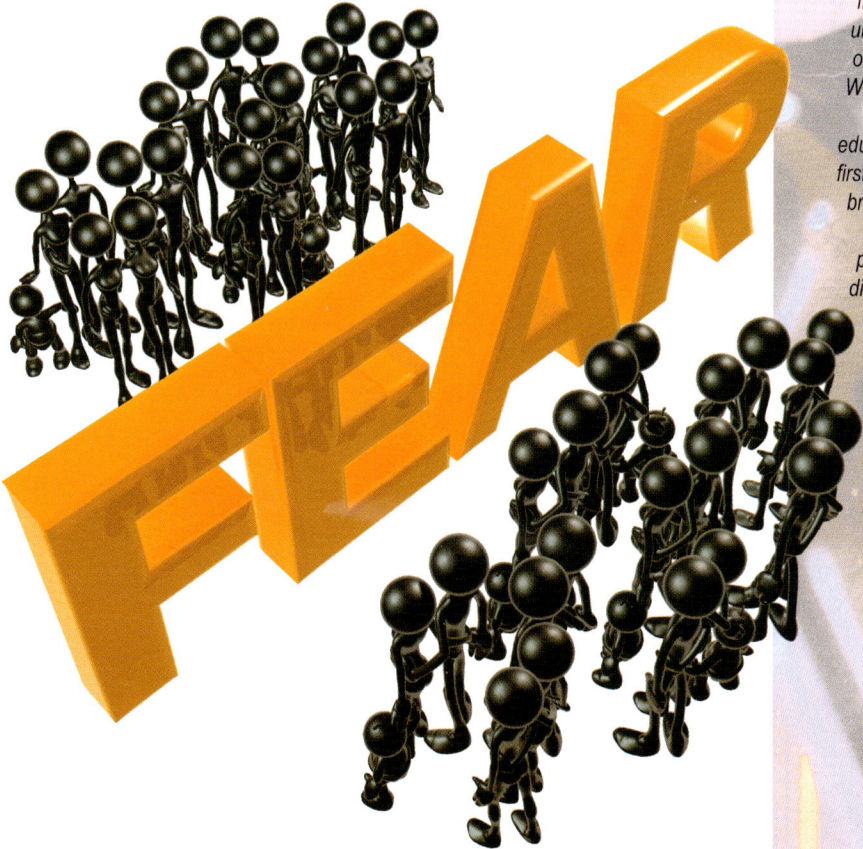

Fear is often at the root of discrimination, and fear generally springs from a lack of understanding or knowledge. When it comes to AIDS, education is the first step toward breaking down the walls of prejudice and discrimination.

The HIV virus is a tiny organism that needs a host cell in order to act like a living thing. Unlike most living things, viruses have no cells. Instead, they are made mostly of genetic material that changes the cells they infect.

cation, but many communities in developing nations are too poor to have school buildings, teachers, and supplies. If schools do exist, they are not always well attended, since children are needed to help their parents provide for the family so that they can survive.

Often, HIV/AIDS education relies on certain community members and organizations that give information and resources to other people. If many people in a country cannot read or write, these community leaders are hard to find. International organizations such as the UN have tried to solve this problem by sending people from other countries into developing countries to teach the people there about HIV/AIDS. Some regions are isolated and hard to reach, and not everyone has access to technology

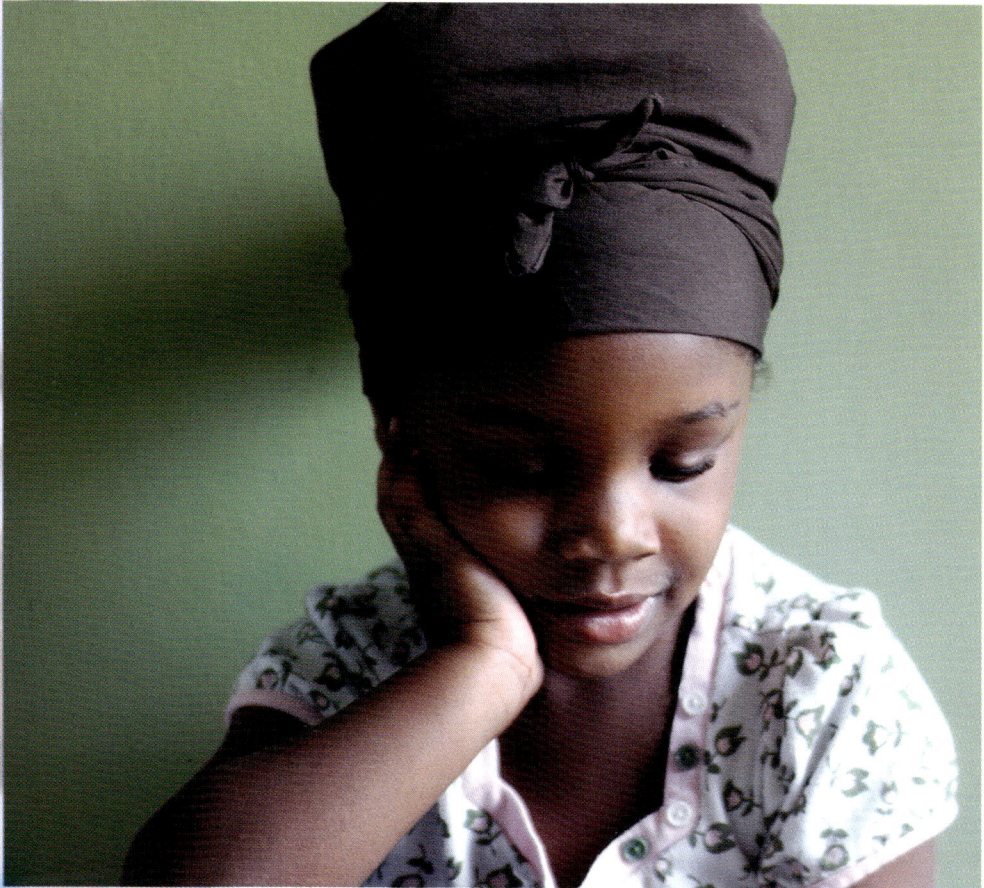

such as the Internet, televisions, and telephones. Many remote communities speak their own dialects, which can make communication difficult. And yet no community is so isolated that it has not been touched by HIV/AIDS!

International intervention and humanitarian efforts face other challenges as well: the foreigners who go into other countries are often seen as intruders who do not fully understand the local culture. For example, if an American tried to teach people in a traditionally conservative country about HIV/AIDS and then distributed condoms, people might be appalled that a foreigner was discussing sex so openly. Imagine how your parents might feel if someone from another country showed up at your school and started passing out things related to unfamiliar sexual practices!

A possible solution to this problem is to train locals to teach their fellow citizens, which would lessen the impression that Westerners are trying to force their culture on other peoples. Even so, effective HIV/AIDS education requires that people openly discuss sex and drug use. While the Western world's media portrays sex fairly openly, and Western fashions for women's clothing are often somewhat revealing, women in many countries are not allowed to show any skin at all and people can be executed for having premarital sex. Imagine how scary it would be to try to talk about and distribute condoms in a country if you knew that you could be killed for doing so! As a result, despite the fact that developing countries have the most need for HIV/AIDS education, they often receive the least.

Politics of Medicine and Treatment Rights

Throughout the world, the controversies surrounding HIV/AIDS also impact the treatment rights of patients. People who are receiving drug treatment for HIV/AIDS must continue taking medication indefinitely. The most

Did You Know?

It is estimated that 12 million children have been orphaned in Africa because their parents died from AIDS.

Real People

When Nosi, a woman living in Port Elizabeth, South Africa, found out that she was pregnant, she knew that she should get tested for HIV. An ex-boyfriend had previously told her that he was HIV-positive, but she kept postponing the test because she was afraid of the results. Her pregnancy convinced her to take the test, because she knew that she would have to take extra precautions for her baby.

On December 15, 2001, Nosi was told that she was HIV-positive. She was initially depressed and felt desperate, but she pressed on for the sake of her unborn child. She would talk to the baby while she was pregnant, apologizing for bringing him into a world at such a great risk. When her son was tested, however, he was HIV-negative.

Despite this good news, Nosi's relationships have not been easy since her diagnosis. When she told her baby's father that he should get tested, he was in denial. He tested positive for HIV, and he descended into a reckless, depressed lifestyle. Nosi and the baby's father broke up because of his alcohol abuse.

Fortunately, Nosi finally found someone who will accept her for who she is. When she met her current love interest, she immediately told him that she was HIV-positive. He accepted this fact and loves her regardless of the disease. Although she wants to marry him, she is afraid to have children with him because of the risks of them contracting HIV. Wherever their relationship goes, Nosi knows that it is possible to find love even if she is HIV-positive.

common treatment to keep HIV patients healthy involves a "cocktail," or combination, of many different pills. Taking so much medicine every day and visiting a doctor so often costs a lot of money.

People in developed countries usually have access to *antiretroviral* treatment. Such medicines have been available to people in Western countries since the mid-1990s. These drugs are usually taken as part of combination therapy, and the term **Highly Active Antiretroviral Therapy** (HAART) refers to a combination of three or more anti-HIV drugs. This treatment consists of a variety of drugs that prevent the replication of the HIV virus. By preventing the onset of AIDS, the treatment can help keep an HIV-positive person relatively healthy for years. Although this treatment is usually effective, it only lasts as long as the patient takes the pills every day for the rest of her life.

Treatment is difficult enough in developed countries—imagine having to take handfuls of pills every day for the rest of your life!—but it is impossible in areas where the medicines are not even available. People who cannot afford enough food for their families can hardly be expected to pay for multiple medications every day for the rest of their lives.

Mothers with HIV can reduce the risk of transmitting the virus to their babies by taking a long course of antiretroviral medications and avoiding breastfeeding—but breastfeeding is the cheapest way for a poor woman to feed her child. What's more, many pregnant women in developing countries do not have access to these antiretroviral drugs. This is why nearly half a million children under the age of fifteen become infected with HIV every year, mostly from mother-to-child transmission.

The problem is so severe that, at the September 22, 2003 UN General Assembly Meeting on HIV/AIDS, representatives from WHO, UNAIDS, and the Global Fund declared the lack of access to HIV treatment a global health emergency. Although the number of people receiving necessary treatment has increased since then,

Did You Know?

In developing countries, 7.1 million people are in immediate need of AIDS drugs to save their lives, but only 2.015 million of them (28%) are currently receiving those medications.

People who do medical research must be paid; the equipment is expensive; and the materials are often costly as well. All this means that research requires a lot of money to keep it going. Meanwhile, politicians are pressured by many other interests that also require funding. It is difficult for government leaders to know which interest is the priority.

the problem remains. There is currently a campaign called "All by 2010," which refers to the goal of providing universal access to antiretroviral treatment by the year 2010. Universal access will be achieved when 80 percent of all people in urgent need of treatment are receiving it. International organizations, such as the UN and nongovernment organizations, have been trying to implement programs that will help people in developing countries access the necessary treatment.

As it stands today, the world is far from reaching that goal. These efforts take money—and the politics of the world are influenced by big businesses that direct money toward their own interests. Other smaller problems may seem more pressing to those who are not dying of AIDS, and these problems also require money. In the competi-

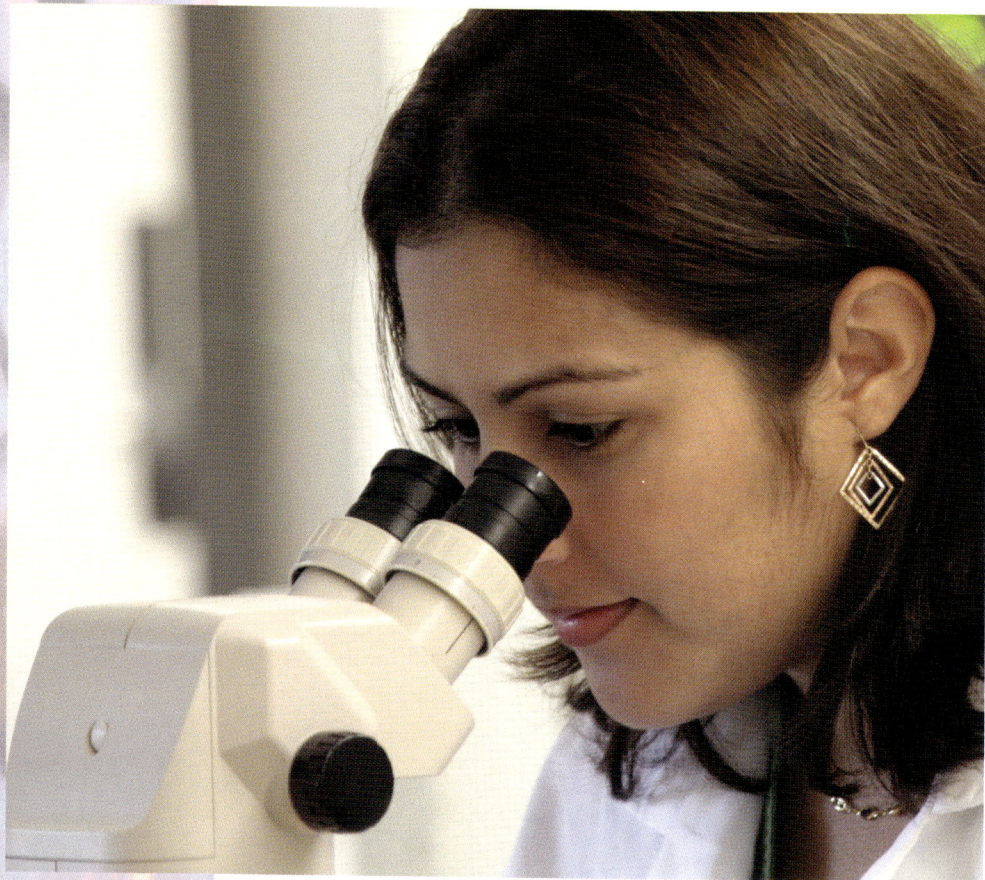

tion for the world's dollars, AIDS—and its victims—often loses.

Politics of Research

Meanwhile, even for those who have money for the current HIV medications, these medicines can only prolong the onset of AIDS, not prevent it entirely. Researchers are working to find more effective treatments and potentially a cure for HIV/AIDS; they are also working on an HIV vaccine. Other diseases caused by viruses have been virtually eliminated through the development of vaccinations, and scientists are hopeful that they will one day find the answer to HIV as well.

However, this research is expensive and time-consuming. Skilled doctors could spend their lifetimes trying to find new developments in the fight against HIV/AIDS, but they might not be among the lucky few who actually make a breakthrough. Governments are reluctant to invest money into research if they are not guaranteed results.

Effective medical research also requires that treatments be tested on people. The ethics of medical testing have been debated, because people who volunteer to be in the test group could experience dangerous side effects and even die. Without this test group, however, it is impossible to be positive that the treatment is effective and safe. Even if a researcher were to develop what he or she believes to be a brilliant new treatment for HIV, pharmaceutical companies would not market it unless it was proven to be safe.

As researchers struggle for funding and support, HIV/AIDS patients are left waiting for better treatment. Around the world, nations, organizations, and individuals are asking the question: Where do we go from here?

Ask the Doctor

Q: I am HIV-positive, and I am pregnant. What should I do? I don't want to bring a child into the world if he or she is also going to be HIV-positive.

Don't worry—with proper precautions, it is possible that your child will not be HIV-positive. You should first tell your doctor so that you can be prescribed a series of antiretroviral medications. Try to stay healthy during your pregnancy, and make sure that you take these medicines. Your doctor might talk to you about other options to reduce the risk of your child contracting HIV. Once you give birth, do not breastfeed the baby. You can find baby formula in most grocery stores, and many varieties ensure that your baby will have adequate nutrition without the HIV-related risks of breast-feeding. With the help of your doctor, you can have a healthy child.

STRAIGHT FROM THE SOURCE
The Ethics of Research

(From N. A. Christakis, L.A. Lynn, and A. Castelo, International Conference on AIDS, June 1991)

The AIDS pandemic has called into question the basing of clinical research ethics on Western ideals alone. Certain research protocols involving consenting adults that are unacceptable in some countries may be acceptable in others. A proposed Brazilian study is illustrative. The study is a two-arm, randomized, controlled clinical trial that will compare dideoxycytidine (ddC) with *placebo* in order to assess the relative efficacy of this antiretroviral agent in prolonging survival and improving the quality of life of patients with HIV infection and in order to determine if an investment by the Brazilian government in ddC might ultimately prove cost-saving to society. This study raises two important questions: Is it ethical to conduct a placebo-controlled trial when a drug is known to prolong survival exists? Is it acceptable to design a clinical study to answer an economic question? This trial must be viewed as permissible since the mere existence of an expensive or relatively cost-ineffective drug elsewhere in the world—namely zidovudine, which is available in the developed world—constitutes only theoretical availability in Brazil, where the government does not pay for it at present, where no insurer covers its purchase, and where most patients simply cannot afford it. However, to justify the use of ddC rather than zidovudine as the study drug in this developing world study, two criteria must be met: 1) there must be some expectation that ddC will be clinically effective, and 2) there must be the expectation that ddC would indeed be more cost-effective than both placebo and zidovudine. Two further criteria regarding the trial in general must be met: 1) the trial must be subjected to the review of a local ethics committee, and 2) there must be a prior commitment by the drug manufacturer and the sponsoring government agency to provide ddC to the population should it prove to be clinically active and cost-effective. The abuse of developing world citizens is clearly unacceptable. This case illustrates that ethical decision-making is powerfully influenced by local disease patterns, local values, and local economies. From this cross-cultural perspective, clinical research that does not harm patients, that provides a meaningful benefit to them, and that is aimed at obtaining economic data that will determine drug availability is acceptable and indeed necessary.

What Do You Think?

- Does the author make a good case for medical research regarding HIV/AIDS? What are the reasons given in favor of this research?

- In your opinion, are the risks of these tests worth the potential benefits of the treatments?

- Should governments fund HIV/AIDS research? In your opinion, what percentage of the national budget should be given to this specific cause?

- Would you ever volunteer to be in a test group for medical research? Why or why not?

Find Out More

For more information about current issues involving HIV/ AIDS, check out these Web sites:

HIV and AIDS information from an international AIDS charity
www.avert.org

HIV/AIDS Resources
www.thebody.com

Here's what you need to know

- Current HIV/AIDS campaigns have given individuals greater ability to make a difference.
- It can often be difficult for politicians to focus on a specific problem because people within governments have different opinions and many responsibilities.
- NGOs (nongovernment organizations) usually focus on specific issues and can be effective by themselves, but they also petition governments for legislation.
- Average consumers in developed countries can help the fight against HIV/AIDS just by purchasing certain products, since many companies are donating a portion of profits to HIV/AIDS programs.

Words to Understand

A *nongovernment organization* is a group created by private people (those who are acting out of their personal interests instead of representing voters) without any government participation or representation.

Activism is action taken by humans in support of or against a particular cause.

Initiatives are the first steps in a plan or task.

Consumption is, in economic terms, the act of buying goods and services that have value.

6
Where Do We Go from Here?

Clearly, a lot of work still needs to be done before HIV/ AIDS is eliminated from our world. Researchers are hard at work trying to find new, improved methods of treatment for patients, but people continue to be diagnosed with and die from HIV/AIDS every day. Governments, *nongovernment organizations*, and individuals around the world are trying to find the best ways to raise money for research and distribute resources to the people who need them the most.

Current trends in HIV/AIDS *activism* have been driven by regular people who want to make a difference. With new campaigns and many organizations through which people can volunteer and donate, individuals no longer have to feel powerless as they hear about more people dying from the disease. HIV/AIDS affects us all in some way—and now we all have opportunities to make a difference in our own communities and in the world, through these new projects.

Nongovernment Organizations and Activism

When governments and international organizations such as the UN try to take charge of *initiatives*, they often struggle with diverse opinions. Politicians have to sort through many issues and influences in order to make decisions. Sometimes, politicians will oppose legislation simply because it was presented by members of the opposing party. Or HIV/AIDS issues may not seem like a priority compared to issues of national security, for example. This means that every government decision has to take many factors into account and go through many steps to achieve the needed funds, because each issue is competing with others to be the top priority. So, although governments usually have the resources and power to make a difference, they are not always efficient.

Nongovernment organizations—NGOs—offer a solution to this dilemma. Since these groups are not affiliated with governments, they do not need to worry about as many technicalities and roadblocks. Also, since they are not in charge of maintaining order for society as a whole, they have the ability to focus on a very specific topic and bring all their energy to bear on it. However, they also do not usually have a large amount of money from which to draw, because they cannot tax citizens like governments can. As a result, many NGOs focus on spreading information and increasing support for a cause so that people will then ask their politicians to institute change.

NGOs vary in their size and resources, from small local organizations to international groups. Many countries have NGOs that focus on the issue of HIV/AIDS in their own country. An example is the Remedios AIDS Foundation, Inc. (HAF) in the Philippines. This organization was started in 1991 and provides services such as counseling, resources, education, and community outreach. RAF has created affiliations with other HIV/AIDS NGOs to

The AIDS Quilt, each panel created by friends and loved ones in memory of a person who died of AIDS, displayed in Washington, D.C. The Quilt has been a visible symbol of loss, and a call to activism, for many people.

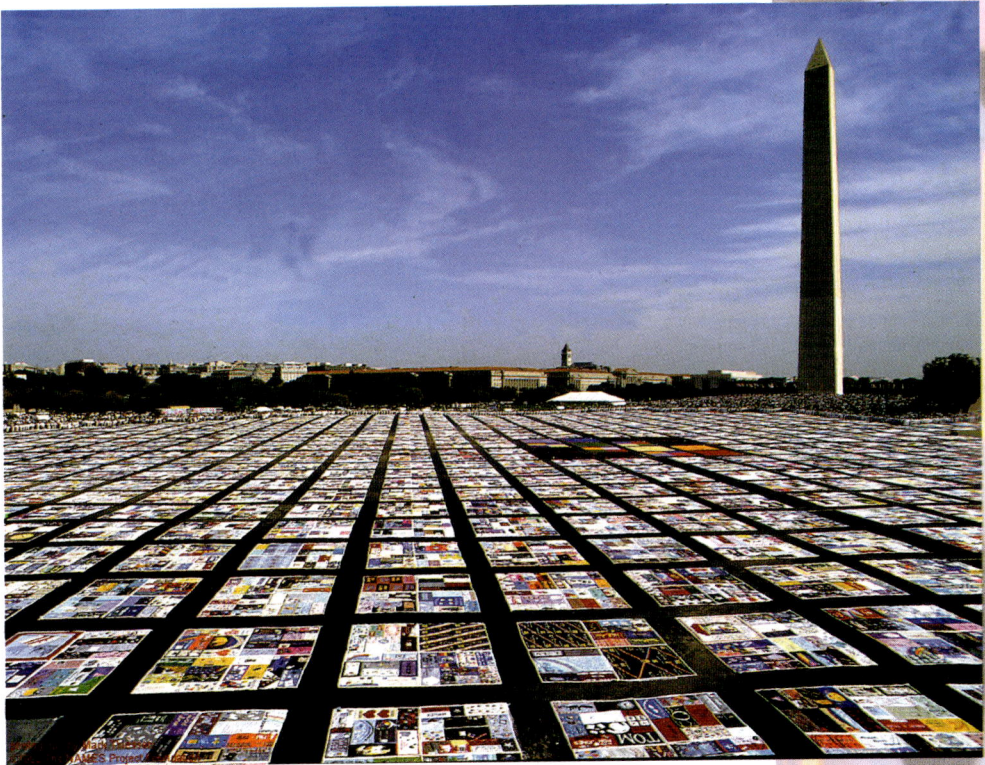

Real People

Anthony J. Raiola did not take the news well that he was HIV-positive. When he was diagnosed in 1996, he saw the disease as an excuse to live recklessly. As he wrote on the Avert Web site, "I was in so much denial I ran the streets as I had before smoking crack and just wanting to get high and higher, because I thought if I was going to die, I was going to die happy and high."

What he did not realize is that an HIV-positive diagnosis is by no means a death sentence. In 2000, after four years of living with the disease, he decided that it was time for him to turn his life around. He got help and overcame his drug addiction, and he sought information about HIV/AIDS.

Now, Anthony helps give other people hope and spreads the message that "WE CAN LIVE." He serves as an HIV/AIDS outreach worker, educator, and test counselor. He has also participated in numerous groups within the New York government, such as the HIV/AIDS Planning Council, Advisory Group to the Planning Council, HIV/AIDS Advocate, and Human and Civil Rights Advocate.

Oddly, his diagnosis eventually helped Anthony find his passion in life. He writes, "I have never been more content and happy than now."

increase awareness of the disease and prevention methods. In the United States, meanwhile, the Henry J. Kaiser Family Foundation has been a leader in major health care issues such as HIV/AIDS. The Kaiser Family Foundation runs its own research and communications programs so that all people, including politicians, will have access to the latest information about HIV/AIDS and other health issues. This foundation has recently been increasingly involved in global health issues as well.

Amnesty International is a well-known and powerful NGO that fights for human rights for all people. Although its mission is much broader than many NGOs, it also campaigns for improved availability of HIV/AIDS treatment and education for all people. Poor people have the same human rights as wealthy members of society, but they are not given the same access to medications they need for survival. Due to this inequality, Amnesty asks people to write to their representatives and urge them to pass legislation that will distribute resources and medications to HIV-positive people around the world. This relationship is common, where NGOs focus on a cause and try to gain support and resources from governments. Therefore, individuals and regular citizens can impact legislation and make HIV/AIDS a priority for politicians.

World AIDS Day 2006
November 30th, 2006

Did You Know?

As of September 2007, the Global Fund finances had provided 1.4 million people with treatment for HIV/AIDS and 33.5 million people with voluntary HIV testing!

World AIDS Day is observed on December 1 each year. (Shown here is the logo for the 2006 observance.) The concept of a World AIDS Day originated at the 1998 World Summit of Ministers of Health on Programmes for AIDS Prevention. Since then, it has been taken up by governments, international organizations, and charities around the world.

Change through Consumption

Since one of the largest issues facing HIV/AIDS activism is global inequality, new projects are trying to encourage people in developed countries to contribute to funds through their everyday activities. Obviously, people with more money tend to buy more goods. This explains why people in developed countries consume, or purchase, more than people in developing countries who might hardly have enough money for food.

A significant portion of the money people spend every month goes toward new clothes. Acknowledging this trend, fashion designers, companies, and celebrities have been teaming with HIV/AIDS activists to create new products. Usually, a portion of the profits made from the sale of the products is donated to HIV/AIDS research and distribution of medical supplies and resources to areas with the greatest need.

The most successful of these campaigns has been (PRODUCT) RED. This campaign is a collaboration of different companies and manufacturers to help distribute antiretroviral medications to HIV-positive people in Africa. Companies agree to offer a product that is designated as (RED), such as a Gap fashion item or a specific Razr cell phone from Motorola. Other products from various manufacturers include (RED) credit cards, shoes, and computers. Although not all of these products are actually red in color, they are all designated (RED) so that consumers know that they are helping fight HIV/AIDS. When these products are purchased, a percentage of the profits is given to the Global Fund.

The Global Fund was established in 2002 with the support of global leaders and former UN Secretary General Kofi Annan. Its purpose is to increase resources to fight

Ask the Doctor

Q: I recently performed oral sex on my boyfriend, and he was not wearing a condom. Could I get HIV from this?

Although the risk is estimated to be lower than having unprotected anal or vaginal sex, it is possible to contract HIV through oral sex. The risk increases if the person giving the oral sex has open cuts or sores in his or her mouth. There is also a greater chance of transmission if the person receiving oral sex ejaculates in the partner's mouth. This is why condoms should be worn if a male is receiving oral sex, and females should wear a latex barrier if they are receiving oral sex. In any case, it is always important to know and trust your partner.

AIDS, tuberculosis, and malaria. It relies on local owner-ship, so that countries can design and establish their own programs. The Global Fund has selected specific, effective programs and grants to receive funds through (PROD-UCT) RED. Since the campaign began, (RED) partners have generated more than $60 million for the Global Fund.

Other companies have helped in the fight against HIV/AIDS by donating a portion of profits to the cause. In February 2008, the fashion store H&M partnered with Designers Against AIDS (DAA) to sell a line of clothes called "Fashion Against AIDS." DAA is a nonprofit orga-nization that seeks to influence public opinion and spread awareness by collaborating with fashion designers, musi-cians, and other artists. In this campaign, celebrity music artists such as Timbaland, Rihanna, and My Chemical Romance designed clothing free of charge. When these clothes are purchased at H&M stores, 25 percent of the selling price is donated to HIV/AIDS programs around the world. With the success of these *consumption* cam-paigns, hopefully more corporations will join the fight against HIV/AIDS.

These and other projects are helping give HIV/AIDS patients hope for a future. But this problem is still too big for the politicians, too big for any organization. It needs people around the globe to get involved, so that enormous changes can be achieved. It needs you!

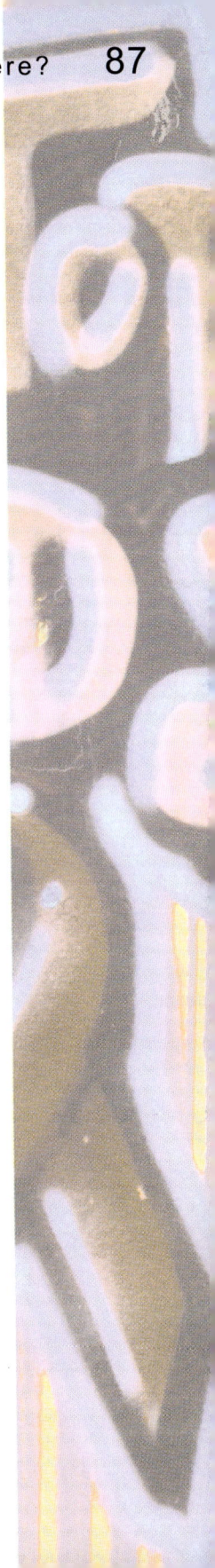

STRAIGHT FROM THE SOURCE
South Africa: "I Am at the Lowest End of All"

(From Amnesty International Document, March 27, 2008)

South Africa is continuing to experience a severe HIV epidemic in which five and a half million South Africans are HIV-infected, one of the highest numbers in the world. Fifty-five per cent of these are women. At the same time South Africa has high levels of sexual and other forms of gender-based violence. In South Africa, women under 25 are three to four times more likely to be HIV-infected than men in the same age group. Women are biologically more vulnerable than men to contracting the virus through unprotected intercourse. They are also placed at risk of infection through rape, or over time when living in abusive relationships because men who are perpetrators of violence are more likely to engage in risk-taking behaviour themselves.

The discriminatory impact of gender roles and stereotypes can also hamper women's ability to protect themselves and to make the best decisions for their health. For instance, they are often unable to insist on condom use to protect themselves against the risk of HIV transmission by a male partner because they are economically and socially dependent on that partner or his family, and/or because they risk being subjected to violence or abandonment as a result of suggesting condom use. These patterns of discrimination also place women at risk of violence, abandonment and other abuses when they test for HIV and disclose their status. Finally, rural women are disproportionately represented among the poor and unemployed in South Africa. Poverty acts as a barrier to access to health services for rural women living with HIV and AIDS because of distance and the cost of transport, particularly where facilities equipped to provide necessary treatment and care are mainly at hospital level, as opposed to at more accessible local-level clinics. This is particularly a problem in Mpumalanga, one of South Africa's nine provinces.

What Do You Think?

- Why does HIV/AIDS bring up human rights issues?

- Why are women at a greater risk for mistreatment and contracting HIV in South Africa?

- How are these risks increased for rural women? What are some possible solutions to this problem?

- How do you think Amnesty International and other organizations should help solve this problem?

Find Out More

For more information on current HIV/AIDS activism, visit these Web sites:

The Henry J. Kaiser Family Foundation Website
www.kff.org

Product (RED) Official Website
www.joinred.org

For More Information on HIV/AIDS

Books

Flanagan, Wendy. *I Am HIV-Positive.* Portsmouth, N.H.: Heinemann, 2003.

Gallant, Joel. 100 *Questions and Answers About HIV and AIDS.* New York: Jones & Bartlett, 2007.

Hinds, Maurene J. *Fighting the AIDS and HIV Epidemic: A Global Battle.* Berkeley Heights, N.J.: Enslow, 2007.

McFarlane, Katerine. *AIDS: Perspectives.* New York: Greenhaven, 2007.

McIntosh, Kenneth. *Living with the Diagnosis: Youth with HIV/AIDS.* Philadelphia: Mason Crest, 2007.

Stine, Gerald. *AIDS Update 2008.* New York: McGraw-Hill, 2008.

Wagner, Viqi. *AIDS: Opposing Viewpoints.* New York: Greenhaven, 2007.

Whiteside, Alan. *HIV/AIDS: A Very Short Introduction.* New York: Oxford University Press, 2008.

Web Sites

AEGIS (AIDS Educational Global Information System)
www.aegis.com

AIDS Info from the U.S. Department of Health and Human Services
www.aidsinfo.nih.gov

AIDSMAP
www.aidsmap.com

AVERT
www.avert.org/aids.htm

The Body: The Complete HIV/AIDS Resource
www.thebody.com

CDC HIV/AIDS Factsheets
www.cdc.gov/hiv/resources/factsheets

HIV InSite (online textbook from the University of
California)
hivinsite.ucsf.edu/InSite

Kaiser Family Foundation Daily HIV/AIDS Report
www.kff.org/hivaids/

Kids' Health: HIV and AIDS
www.kidshealth.com/teen/sexual_health/stds/std_hiv.
html

Mayo Clinic HIV/AIDS
www.mayoclinic.com/health/hiv-aids/DS00005

Medical News Today: HIV & AIDS
www.medicalnewstoday.com/sections/hiv-aids

MedlinePlus
www.medlineplus.gove

Tufts School of Medicine, Nutrition and AIDS
www.tufts.edu/med/nutrition-infection/hiv/

United Nations Development Programme on HIV/
AIDS
www.undp.org/hiv

WHO and AIDS
www.who.int/hiv/en

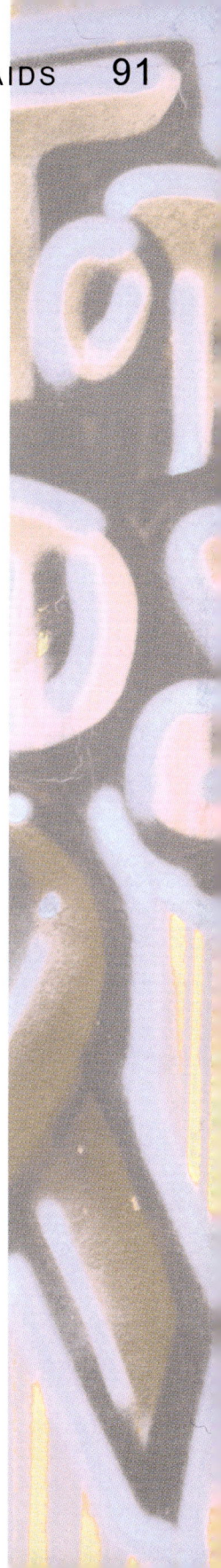

Glossary of HIV/AIDS–Related Terms

When you're reading about HIV/AIDS—or if someone you know has this disease—you may encounter lots of unfamiliar medical terms. This glossary can help you better understand this complicated disease and its treatments.

Acquired Immunity
The body's ability to fight a specific infection, which can be acquired by having and recovering from an infection, by being vaccinated against an infection, or by receiving antibodies through breast milk.

Acquired Immunodeficiency Syndrome (AIDS)
A disease of the body's immune system caused by HIV (human immunodeficiency virus) that leaves the body vulnerable to life-threatening conditions such as infections and cancer.

Acute HIV Infection
The period of rapid growth of the virus during the two to four weeks after HIV infection. Some (but not all) people will experience flu-like symptoms during this period, which can include fever, sore throat, inflamed lymph nodes, and a rash, lasting from a few days to a few weeks.

AIDS-Defining Condition
Any of a list of 26 illnesses that lead to a diagnosis of AIDS when occurring in a person with HIV. Included in the list are Kaposi's sarcoma, pneumocystis, recurrent pneumonia, pulmonary tuberculosis, invasive cervical cancer, and wasting syndrome.

AIDS-Related Cancer
One of the several cancers that are more common or more aggressive in people with HIV, including lymphomas, Kaposi's sarcoma, and cancers that affect the anus and the cervix.

AIDS-Related Complex

A group of conditions that often occur during the early stage of HIV infection, which can include recurrent fevers, unexplained weight loss, diarrhea, herpes, swollen lymph nodes, or fungal infection in the mouth and throat.

Antibody

Also known as immunoglobulin, a protein produced by the body's immune system that recognizes and fights germs and other foreign substances that enter the body.

Antigen

Anything that stimulates the body to produce antibodies to fight it, including bacteria, viruses, and pollen.

Antiretroviral

A medicine that interferes with the ability of a retrovirus (such as HIV) to make more copies of itself.

B-Cell Lymphoma

A type of cancer in the lymphatic tissue, to which people with HIV are more prone.

B Lymphocytes

Also known as B cells, these infection-fighting white blood cells develop in the bone marrow and spleen; in people with HIV, B lymphocytes' ability to do their job is damaged.

Branched Chain DNA Assay (bDNA Assay)

A test that measures a person's viral load (level of HIV present in the blood) to diagnose HIV and monitor disease progression, as well as treatment effectiveness.

Candidiasis

An infection caused by a yeast-like fungus that produces white patches on the skin, nails, and mucus membranes. It is considered an AIDS-defining condition in people with HIV.

Cardiomyopathy
A condition that weakens the heart muscle, which can cause irregular heartbeat and decreased heart function. It may occur in people with HIV.

CD4 Cell
Also known as helper T cell, these infection-fighting white blood cells signal the other cells in the immune system to do their jobs. The number of CD4 cells in a blood sample indicates how healthy the person's immune system is. HIV infects and kills CD4 cells.

CD4 Cell Count
Measuring the number of CD4 cells in a blood sample is one of the most useful ways to tell how far HIV/AIDS has progressed. Health-care providers use this count to determine when to begin or stop therapies and to measure response to treatments. A normal CD4 cell count is between 500 and 1,400 cells per cubic millimeter of blood. When an individual with HIV has a CD4 cell count at or below 200, he is considered to have AIDS.

CD8 Cell
Also called killer T cell, this is a type of white blood cell that is able to recognize and kill cells that are infected by a foreign invader.

Cervical Cancer
A condition in which a cancerous growth forms on the lower portion of the uterus, which is called the cervix; it is a type of cancer to which people with HIV/AIDS are more susceptible.

CIPRA (Comprehensive International Program on Research on AIDS)
A program run by the U.S. NIAID (National Institute on Allergy and Infectious Diseases) to support research and affordable treatment of HIV/AIDS in poor countries.

CMV (cytomegalovirus)
An infectious eye disease that is the most common cause of blindness in people with HIV.

Co-Infection
Infection with more than one germ at a time; for example, a person with HIV may also be infected with hepatitis C or tuberculosis (TB).

Combination Therapy
When two or more drugs are used together to treat HIV, which has proven to be more effective than using a single drug.

Contagious
When a disease passes easily between people through normal day-to-day contact. HIV is not contagious.

Cryptoccocis
An infection caused by a fungus that enters the body through the lungs and usually spreads to the brain. It is considered an AIDS-defining condition in people with HIV.

DNA (deoxyribonucleic acid)
Chemical structure that contains the genetic instructions for reproduction within all cells.

ELISA (enzyme-linked immunosorbent assay)
A sensitive laboratory test used to determine the presence of antibodies to HIV in the blood or saliva. Positive ELISA results should always be confirmed with another test called a Western blot.

End-Stage Disease
The final phase in the course of a disease that will lead to the person's death.

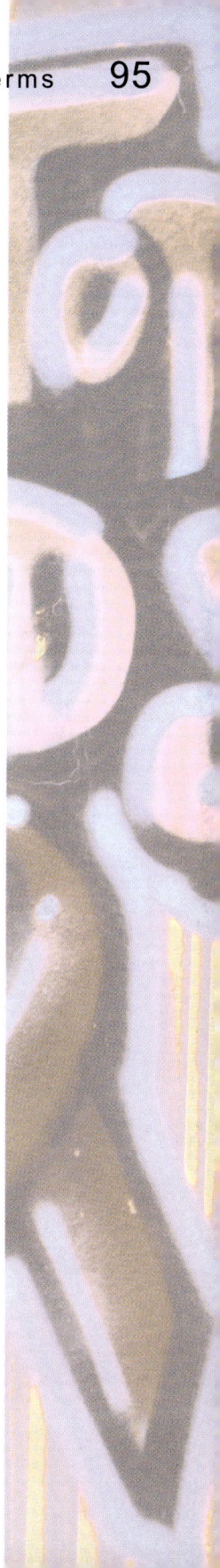

Entry Inhibitors
A class of anti-HIV drugs designed to interfere with HIV's ability to enter a host cell through the cell's surface.

Envelope
The outer protective membrane of HIV cells. Proteins in the envelope allow HIV to attach to and enter host cells.

Enzyme
A protein in the body that helps a chemical reaction happen.

Fusion Inhibitors
A class of anti-HIV drugs that gets in the way of HIV's outer envelope fusing with a host cell's membrane, thus preventing infection of the cell.

GART (genotypic antiretroviral resistance test) or Genotypic Assay
A test that determines if HIV is resistant to a particular drug. The test uses a blood sample to see if any genetic mutations are present that are associated with resistance to specific drugs.

HAART (highly active antiretroviral therapy)
Treatment regimens that aggressively suppress HIV from copying itself and thus slow the progression of HIV disease. It usually combines three or more anti-HIV drugs.

Helper T Cells
See CD4 Cell

Hemophilia
A hereditary blood defect, occurring almost exclusively in males, characterized by delayed clotting, which can lead to uncontrolled bleeding, even after minor cuts. Because hemophiliacs often receive blood transfusions to treat injuries, they were exposed to HIV during the 1970s, before doctors realized that the blood supply was infected.

HIV (human immunodeficiency virus)
The virus that causes AIDS.

HIV-1
The type of HIV responsible for most of the HIV infections around the world.

HIV-2
A virus that is closely related to HIV-1, which also causes AIDS. Although the two viruses are very similar, immunodeficiency seems to develop more slowly and to be milder in people who have HIV-2. Most people who have HIV-2 live in West Africa. Drugs used to treat HIV-1 are not always effective against HIV-2.

Immune Response
The body's reaction to a foreign invader, such as a bacteria, virus, or fungus.

Immune System
The cells and organs in the body, including the thymus, spleen, lymph nodes, B and T cells, and antigen-presenting cells, whose job is to protect the body against foreign invaders.

Immunocompromised
Unable to mount a normal immune response because of a damaged immune system.

Immunodeficiency
Unable to produce normal amounts of antibodies and/or immune cells.

Immunoglobulin (IG)
See **Antibody**.

Immunosuppression
Inability of the immune system to function normally (which can be caused by treatments such as chemotherapy or by certain diseases such as HIV).

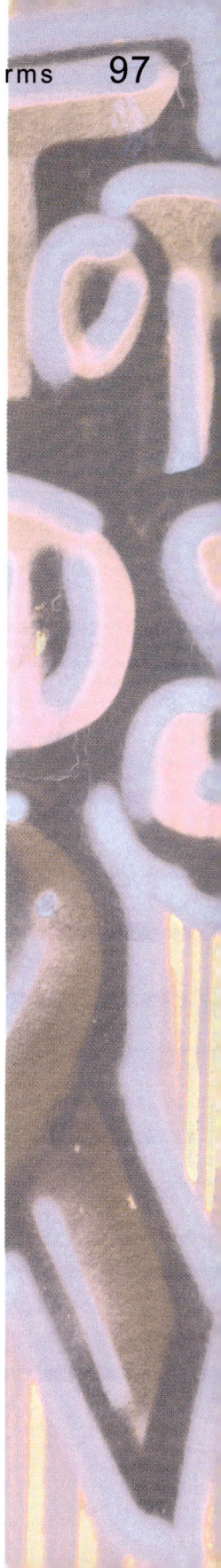

Immunotherapy
Treatment to stimulate or restore the body's ability to fight off diseases.

Incubation Period
The time between when a germ enters the body and when the person develops symptoms.

Infectious
Capable of causing infection.

Integrase
An HIV protein that inserts the virus' genetic information into the infected cell.

Integrase Inhibitors
A class of anti-HIV drugs that prevents the integrase protein from inserting genetic information into the host cell.

Integration
The process by which HIV integrase inserts the virus' genetic material into a host cell.

Interleukin-2 (IL-2)
A protein that helps regulate the immune system by increasing the production of certain disease-fighting white blood cells. HIV infection reduces IL-2 levels, but a man-made version of IL-2 is being researched as a way to treat people with HIV.

Interleukin-7 (IL-7)
Another protein that regulates the immune system by increasing the body's production of certain white blood cells. Man-made IL-7 is used to treat HIV because it makes HIV copy itself in infected cells that are resting, allowing anti-retroviral drugs to target HIV in those cells.

Investigational Drug
Also known as an experimental drug, these medicines' safety and effectiveness have not yet been thoroughly tested.

Kaposi's Sarcoma (KS)
A type of cancer caused by an overgrowth of blood vessels, causing pinkish-purple bumps or spots on the skin. These can also occur inside the body, especially in the intestines, lungs, and lymph nodes, and when this happens, the condition can become life-threatening. KS is considered an AIDS-defining condition. A virus called Kaposi's sarcoma herpesvirus (KSHV) or human herpesvirus 8 often accompanies Kaposi's sarcoma.

Killer T Cell
See **CD8 Cell**.

Latency
The time during which an infection is present within the body without producing any noticeable symptoms. Latency may last for a few years with an HIV infection.

Lentivirus
In Latin, *lente* means "slow;" these are viruses that have a long latency period (like HIV).

Lesion
An area on the skin where the tissue is abnormal, such as a sore or an infected patch.

Leukocytosis
An abnormally high white blood cell count, a condition that usually occurs during an infection.

Leukopenia
A lower than normal white blood cell count.

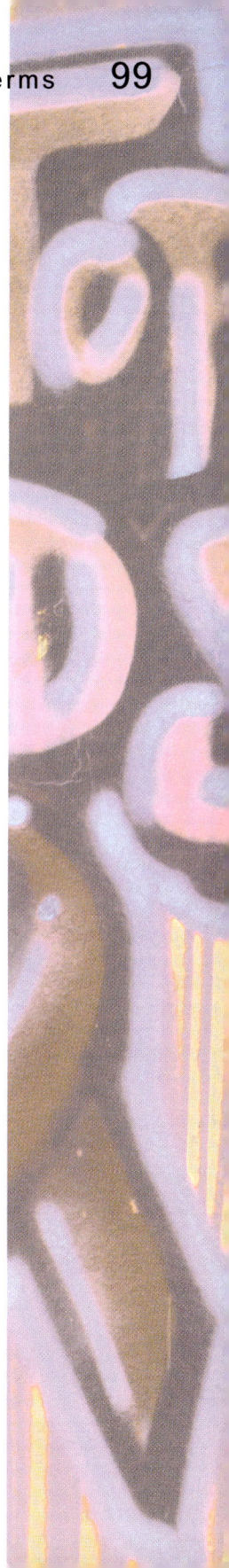

Long-Term Nonprogressors
People who have been infected with HIV for at least 7 years with no symptoms, stable CD4 counts of 600 or more, and no HIV-related diseases.

Lymph
A clear, yellowish fluid that carries white blood cells (which fight disease) from the blood to body tissues.

Lymph Nodes
Small immune system organs that are located throughout the body, where lymph is filtered as it carries white blood cells back from the body tissues to the blood.

Lymphadenopathy Syndrome (LAS)
Swollen and sometimes sore lymph nodes caused by infections (such as HIV, the flu, or mononucleosis) or lymphoma (cancer of the lymph tissue).

Lymphocyte
A type of infection-fighting white blood cell found in the blood and lymph.

Lymphoid Interstitial Pneumonitis (LIP)
A hardening of the parts of the lung that absorb oxygen for which there is no clear treatment. LIP is an AIDS-defining condition in children with HIV.

Lymphokines
Chemical messengers secreted by white blood cells that affect the immune response.

Macrophage
A type of disease-fighting white blood cell that destroys invaders and helps other immune system cells to do their jobs.

Malabsorption Syndrome
When the intestines cannot adequately absorb nutrients. This is a condition that is associated with HIV and that

can lead to loss of appetite, muscle pain, and weight loss.

Memory T Cells

A type of infection-fighting T cell that recognizes foreign invaders it has encountered before (either during an earlier infection or from a vaccination). Memory T cells do their jobs faster and more strongly the second time they see the invader.

Meningitis

Inflammation of the membranes around the brain or spinal cord, which can be caused by bacteria, fungus, or a viral infection like HIV.

Microbes

Living organisms that can only be seen through a microscope, including bacteria, protozoa, viruses, and fungi.

Microsporidiosis

An intestinal infection caused by a parasite that causes diarrhea and loss of weight and strength in people with HIV.

Molluscum Contagiosum

A disease of the skin and mucus membranes that causes white or flesh-colored bumps on the face, neck, hands, underarms, and genitals. A virus causes the condition, but in people with HIV, it usually gets worse with time and does not respond to treatment.

Mucocutaneous

Relating to the mucus membranes and the skin (the eyes, mouth, lips, vagina, and anus, for example).

Mutation

A change or adaptation that can be passed down to future generations. The virus that causes AIDS mutates, which means that an individual strain of HIV can adapt to infect

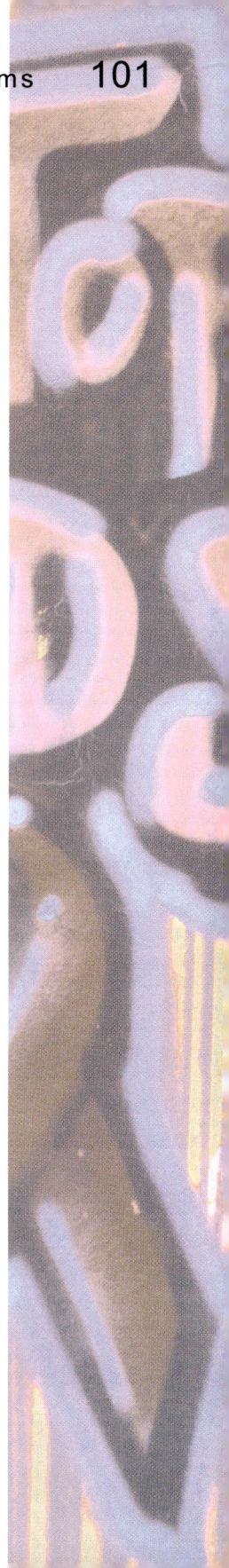

different cell types or to resist certain anti-HIV drugs. Mutations can only occur when the virus is copying itself and not when anti-HIV drugs have suppressed the virus to the point where it is not detectable.

Mycobacterium Avium Complex (MAC)
A life-threatening infection caused by two bacteria found in soil and dust, which is extremely rare in people who do not have HIV. It is considered an AIDS-defining condition in people with HIV.

Myelosuppression
Decreased bone marrow function that means that fewer red blood cells, white blood cells, and platelets (the part of the blood that causes clotting) are produced. It is a side effect of some anti-HIV drugs.

Myopathy
A disease of muscle tissue that can be a side effect of some anti-HIV drugs; HIV itself can also cause it.

Natural Killer Cells (NK cells)
White blood cells that kill tumor cells and other cells infected with viruses or other foreign invaders.

Neuropathy
A disorder caused by damaged nerve cells, which can produce a range of symptoms from a tingly feeling in the toes and fingers to paralysis. Some anti-HIV drugs cause neuropathy, as does HIV itself in some cases.

Neutropenia
A lower than normal number of **neutrophils** in the blood, which can increase the chance of getting bacterial infections. It can be caused by HIV infection, but some anti-HIV drugs also cause it.

Neutrophil
A type of white blood cell that engulfs and kills invaders such as bacteria.

Non-Nucleoside Reverse Transcriptase Inhibitors (NNRTIs)

A kind of anti-HIV drug that binds to and disables the protein that HIV-1 needs to copy itself, bringing an end to HIV-1 multiplication.

Nucleoside

An early version of a nucleotide, the building block that contains DNA and RNA, which are the chemical structures that store the cell's genetic material. Nucleosides must be changed chemically before they can make DNA and RNA.

Nucleoside Analogue Reverse Transcriptase Inhibitor (nuke)

A kind of anti-HIV drug that provides a "bad" version of the building block necessary for HIV reproduction. When it's used instead of a normal nucleoside, reproduction of the virus is halted.

Nucleotide

A building block of the chemical structures (DNA and RNA) that store genetic information within the cell.

Nucleotide Analogue Reverse Transcriptase Inhibitor (nuke)

A kind of anti-HIV drug that provides a "bad" version of a nucleotide, which halts HIV reproduction.

Nukes

See **Nucleoside Analogue Reverse Transcriptase Inhibitor** and **Nucleotide Analogue Reverse Transcriptase Inhibitor.**

Opportunistic Infections (OIs)

Illnesses that occur in people with weakened immune systems, including people with HIV/AIDS. Common OIs in people with AIDS include Pneumocystis carinii pneumonia, histoplasmosis, toxoplasmosis, cryptosporidiosis, and some types of cancers.

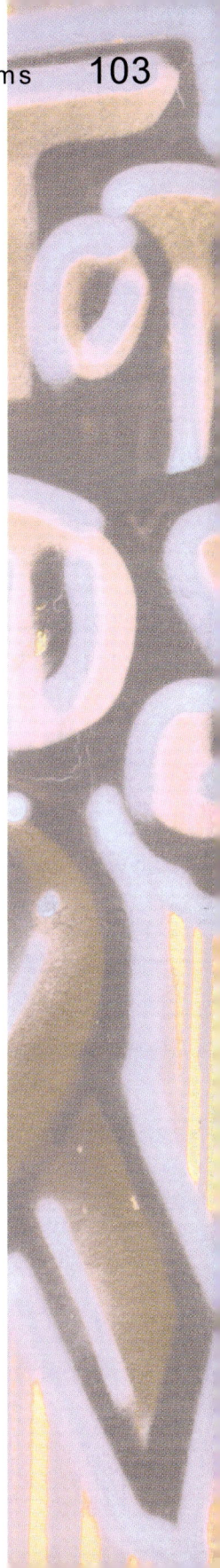

Oral Hairy Leukoplakia (OHL)

A white, hairy, or bumpy patch caused by the Epstein-Barr virus (a member of the herpesvirus family) that appears on the side of the tongue and inside the cheeks, mainly in people with weakened immune systems (including people with HIV).

Osteoporosis

Loss of bone mass, density, and strength, which is usually brought on by old age but can also occur as a result of HIV infection or as a side effect of some anti-HIV drugs.

p24

The protein that surrounds the HIV core where the genetic material is found.

Palliative Care

Medical care that offers no cure but helps reduce the suffering and discomfort caused by the disease's symptoms.

Pancytopenia

A lower than normal level of all types of blood cells, including red blood cells, white blood cells, and platelets.

Paresthesia

Burning, tingling, or pins-and-needles sensations that can be caused as part of neuropathy brought on by certain anti-HIV drugs.

Passive Immunotherapy

A treatment approach that transfers antibodies from one person to another to help the receiver fight infections. An example in HIV treatment is when plasma from healthy HIV-infected people (who have high CD4 counts and high levels of anti-HIV antibodies) is given to people with AIDS who have lost CD4 cells and can no longer make their own antibodies. This treatment has not been very successful with adults, but it is still sometimes used with children who have HIV.

Perinatal Transmission

When a mother with HIV gives her child the virus, either within the womb, during labor and delivery, or through breastfeeding.

Photosensitivity

When skin responds more quickly to sunlight and ultraviolet light, causing sunburns and skin cancer more easily. It can be a side effect of some drugs and can also be caused by HIV infection.

Pill Burden

The number of pills taken each day. A high pill burden may make the person less likely to follow the treatment she needs.

Plasma

The clear, liquid part of the blood in which red blood cells, white blood cells, platelets, nutrients, and wastes are suspended.

Pneumocystis Jiroveci Pneumonia (PCP)

A lung infection that occurs in people with weakened immune systems, including those with HIV, whose first symptoms are difficulty breathing, high fever, and a dry cough. It is considered an AIDS-defining condition in people with HIV.

Post-Exposure Prophylaxis (PEP)

Administration of anti-HIV drugs within 72 hours of a high-risk exposure (such as unprotected sex, needle sharing, or injury) to help prevent HIV infection.

Protease

An enzyme that breaks down proteins into smaller chunks.

Protease Inhibitors (PIs)

A kind of anti-HIV drug that prevents HIV from reproducing by disabling HIV protease.

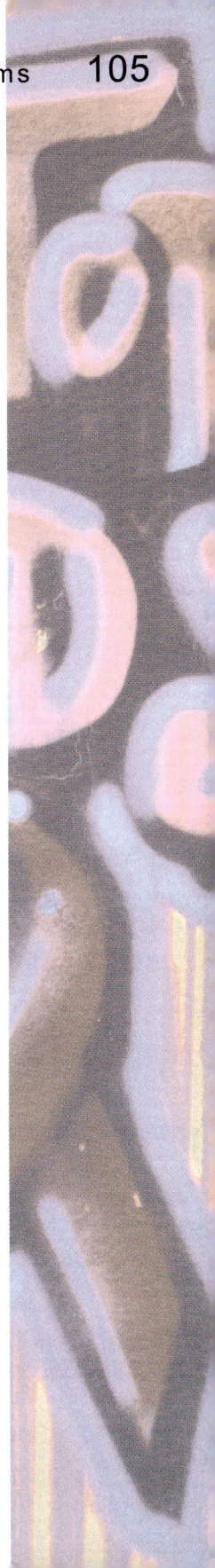

Protease-Sparing Regimen
An anti-HIV drug regimen that does not include a PI.

Protozoa
Tiny, one-celled animals that cause diseases, especially in people with weakened immune systems (including those with HIV). AIDS-defining infections such as toxoplasmosis and cryptosporidiosis are caused by protozoa.

Pulmonary
Having to do with the lungs.

q.d.
Once a day dosing instructions.

q.i.d.
Four times a day dosing instructions.

R5-Tropic Virus
A strain of HIV, also called M-tropic virus.

Receptor
A protein on the surface of a cell that acts as a binding site for substances outside the cell (such as HIV).

Remission
The time during which symptoms diminish or disappear, although the person is still infected.

Retrovirus
A type of virus that stores its genetic information in a single-strand RNA molecule, then builds a double-strand DNA version using an enzyme called reverse transcriptase, which is then integrated into the host cell's own genetic material. HIV is a retrovirus.

Reverse Transcriptase (RT)
An enzyme found in HIV and other retroviruses that converts single-strand RNA into double-strand DNA.

RNA (ribonucleic acid)
The chemical structure that carries genetic instructions for some viruses.

Seborrheic Dermatitis
A skin condition common in people with HIV where the skin is covered with loose, greasy, or dry scales that are white or yellowish. It can occur on the scalp, eyelids, eyebrows, ears, lips, and along any skin folds.

Sepsis
A blood-borne infection, usually caused by bacteria, to which people with HIV are more prone.

Superinfection
A new infection on top of an existing infection, such as when a person with HIV-1 becomes infected with a new strain of HIV. Superinfection makes treatment more challenging.

T Cell
A type of disease-fighting white blood cell, which includes CD4 and CD8 cells. The "T" stands for thymus, where T cells mature.

Therapeutic HIV Vaccine
A vaccine used to treat a person who is already infected with HIV to boost his immune response and better control the virus.

Thymus
An organ behind the breastbone in the chest where infection-fighting T cells develop.

t.i.d.
Three times a day dosing instructions.

Tolerability
How well a medicine can be tolerated—or endured—by a person taking it.

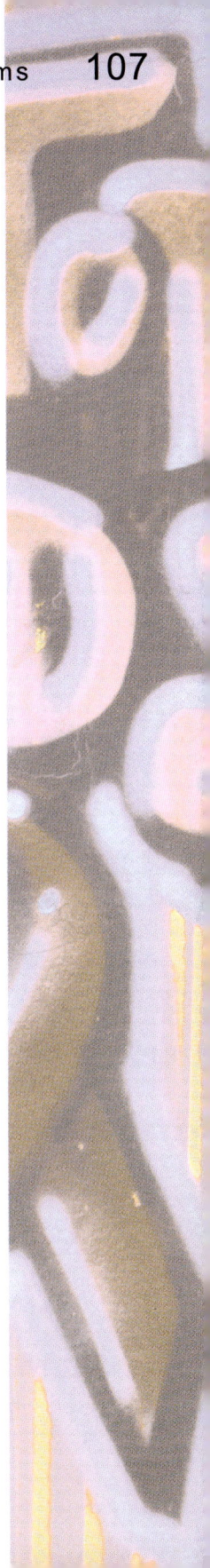

Tolerance
A decreased response to repeated doses of a drug.

Toxoplasmosis
An infection caused by a protozoa that is carried by cats and birds, and is also found in soil contaminated by cat feces and in pork. Toxoplasmosis is an AIDS-defining condition in people with HIV.

Transcription
The step in the HIV life cycle when its DNA is used as a template to create copies of its RNA.

Translation
The step that follows transcription, where the genetic information in the RNA is used to build new copies of HIV.

Vaccine
A substance that stimulates the body's immune response to prevent or control an infection. Researchers are testing vaccines both to prevent and treat HIV/AIDS, but there is currently no approved vaccine.

Viral Load
The amount of HIV RNA in a blood sample, which is an important indicator of the disease's progression.

Virus
A microscopic organism that requires a host cell in order to make more copies of itself. The cold and the flu are both caused by a virus—and so is AIDS.

Western Blot Test
A laboratory technique used to detect HIV proteins in the blood, which is used to confirm a positive ELISA.

Bibliography

American Medical Student Association
www.amsa.org/uhc

The Body
www.thebody.org

CDC
www.cdc.gov

Centers for Medicare and Medicaid Services
www.cms.hhs.gov

H&M Launches "Fashion Against Aids"
w w w . H m . C o m / Q a / F a s h i o n p r e s s r e l e a s e .
Ahtml?Pressreleaseid=545

Health08
www.health08.org/issue_globalhealth_hivaids.cfm

HIV Positive
www.hivpositive.com

(PRODUCT) RED
www.joinred.com

Time Magazine, Profiles of Heroes
www.time.com/time/time100/heroes/profile/milk01.
html

The United Nations
www.un.org/english

U.S. Department of Health and Human Services
www.hhs.gov

World Health Organization
www.who.int/en

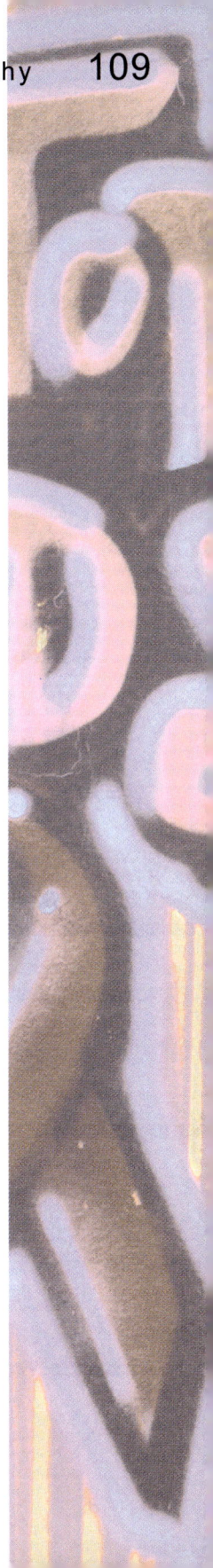

Index

Picture Credits

Dreamstime
  Alinoubigh: p. 17
  Ariy: p. 37
  Bernardo69: p. 64
  Bloopiers: p. 54
  Breathtaking Blue Sky: p. 29
  Caraman: p. 57
  Celsopupo: pp. 8–9
  Dusanzidar: p. 63
  Eliron: p. 18
  Eraxion: pp. 11, 56
  Filtv: p. 58
  Hjalmeida: p. 53
  Icholakov: p. 55
  InFocus: p. 28
  IqSolution: p. 45

Kuzma: p. 61
Lokes: p. 27
Meckfisto: p. 14
Nedens: p. 32
Sebcz: p. 12
SGame: pp. 8–9
Walterq: p. 30

Government of India: p. 43

University of Michigan
  Thom, Robert: p. 47

World Health Organization
  p. 41
  p. 46

To the best knowledge of the publisher, all other images are in the public domain. If any image has been inadvertently uncredited, please notify Harding House Publishing Service, Vestal, New York 13850, so that rectification can be made for future printings.

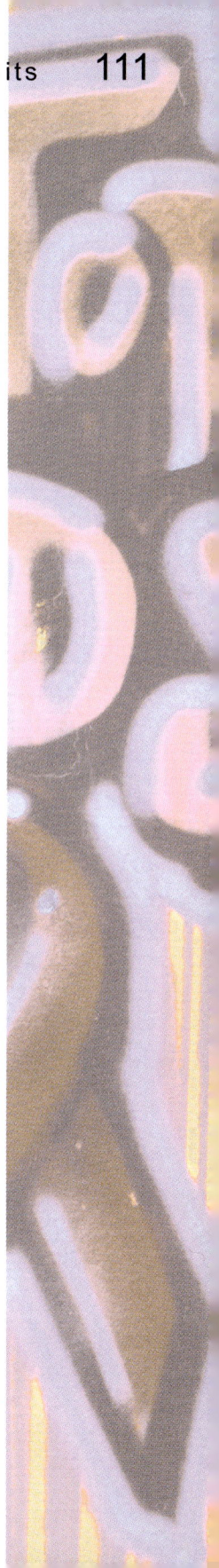

About the Author

Jacquelyn Simone has studied both journalism and politics. She encourages all readers to become involved with HIV/AIDS activism and teach others about the disease.

About the Consultant

Elise DeVore Berlan, MD, MPH, FAAP, is a faculty member of the Division of Adolescent Health at Nationwide Children's Hospital and an Assistant Professor of Clinical Pediatrics at The Ohio State University College of Medicine. She completed her Fellowship in Adolescent Medicine at Children's Hospital Boston and obtained a Master's Degree in Public Health at the Harvard School of Public Health. Dr. Berlan completed her residency in pediatrics at the Children's Hospital of Philadelphia, where she also served an additional year as Chief Resident. She received her medical degree from the University of Iowa College of Medicine. Dr. Berlan is board certified in Pediatrics and board eligible in Adolescent Medicine. She provides primary care and consultative services in the area of Young Women's Health, including gynecological problems, concerns about puberty, reproductive health services, and reproductive endocrine disorders.